AN INTRODUCTION
TO COMMUNICATION
DISORDERS

FORTHCOMING TITLES

Brain Injury Rehabilitation
A neuro-functional approach
Jo Clark-Wilson and Gordon Muir Giles

Writing for Health Professionals
Philip Burnard

Psychology and Counselling for Health Professionals
Edited by Rowan Bayne and Paula Nicholson

Occupational Therapy for Orthopaedic Conditions
Dina Penrose

Living with Continuing Perceptuo-Motor Difficulties
Dorothy E. Penso

Teaching Students in Clinical Settings
Jackie Stengelhofen

Speech and Language Disorders in Children
Dilys A. Treharne

THERAPY IN PRACTICE SERIES
Edited by Jo Campling

This series of books is aimed at 'therapists' concerned with rehabilitation in a very broad sense. The intended audience particularly includes occupational therapists, physiotherapists and speech therapists, but many titles will also be of interest to nurses, psychologists, medical staff, social workers, teachers or volunteer workers. Some volumes are interdisciplinary, others are aimed at one particular profession. All titles will be comprehensive but concise, and practical but with due reference to relevant theory and evidence. They are not research monographs but focus on professional practice, and will be of value to both students and qualified personnel.

An Introduction to Communication Disorders

DIANA SYDER
Lecturer in Speech Pathology and Therapeutics,
University of Sheffield, UK

CHAPMAN & HALL
London · New York · Tokyo · Melbourne · Madras

Published by Chapman & Hall, 2–6 Boundary Row, London SE1 8HN

Chapman & Hall, 2–6 Boundary Row, London SE1 8HN, UK

Blackie Academic & Professional, Wester Cleddens Road, Bishopbriggs, Glasgow G64 2NZ, UK

Chapman & Hall, 29 West 35th Street, New York NY10001, USA

Chapman & Hall Japan, Thomson Publishing Japan, Hirakawacho Nemoto Building, 6F, 1–7–11 Hirakawa-cho, Chiyoda-ku, Tokyo 102, Japan

Chapman & Hall Australia, Thomas Nelson Australia, 102 Dodds Street, South Melbourne, Victoria 3205, Australia

Chapman & Hall India, R. Seshadri, 32 Second Main Road, CIT East, Madras 600 035, India

Distributed in the USA and Canada by Singular Publishing Group Inc., 4284 41st Street, San Diego, California 92105

First edition 1992

© 1992 Chapman & Hall

Typeset in 10/12pt Times by Intype, London
Printed in Great Britain by St Edmundsbury Press Ltd, Bury St Edmunds, Suffolk

ISBN 0 412 38850 2   1 56593 041 X (USA)

A catalogue record for this book is available from the British Library for Dick and Monica

Contents

Acknowledgements

Many thanks are due to colleagues who have willingly provided advice, clinical information and material; specifically to Caroline Pickstone, Isabel O'Leary, Shelagh Brumfitt, Kate Sisum, Alexa Warden, Sarah Howard, Peter Trewhitt and Anne Crichton. I would particularly like to thank Richard Body for his ongoing support and for helping me to refine my own ideas about communication, not to mention his patience and cooperation in the workshops we led together on Communication Disorders.

I thank all the clients who have tolerated my sometimes clumsy efforts on their behalf and allowed me to learn from their experiences.

Preface

I have wanted to write this book since I qualified as a communication therapist and first began to suspect how little other health workers understood about the nature of communication disorders. I also realized how hard this was both on them and on the people in their care.

Despite the fact that the whole field of interpersonal skills has become a rather trendy if esoteric discipline in the last few years, there has not been a subsequent upsurge of interest in the pathology of communication. It surprises me that communication disorders still feature little, if at all, on the undergraduate syllabuses of medical students and nurses. This is despite the fact that these people will have to spend much of their professional lives caring for people who are not able to communicate efficiently or effectively. Even when the same students have reached senior positions in their careers, many will feel ill-equipped to help and frustrated by their failures with such a diverse client group.

This book attempts to bridge a gap between the many general information pamphlets provided by the various charity organizations which have an interest in specific communication disorders and the heavier textbooks aimed at people who already have a background in speech and language pathology. It is intended to be read as a whole and an understanding of the general nature of communication disorders as well as of specific disorders is built up through the text.

The term 'therapist' is used to refer to a communication therapist unless otherwise specified. For years British speech therapists have expressed dissatisfaction with their professional label and the misconceptions it breeds, but until recently they have been unable to agree on a viable alternative. At the time of writing the professional body has just decided to rename its practitioners 'speech and language therapists'. As this represents such a small proportion of therapists world-wide, and at the risk of adding to any confusion, I have decided to use the term communication therapist. It has always seemed the most sensible description to me and it is the one that has currently been adopted for use in the Health Service in Sheffield. Just to complicate the issue further, practitioners in the United States and Australia are known as speech pathologists.

1

Communication: some basic concepts

WHY DO WE COMMUNICATE?

Our desire to express ourselves is powerful and originates from basic drives to satisfy both our physical and emotional needs. It is necessary for us to interact with other human beings for survival, support and stimulation. In fact for emotional health we simultaneously have to do two almost contradictory things. We have to define ourselves as part of a social group and as having things in common with the other members of that group and yet at the same time as individuals having a unique identity. We also need to express our own personality and individuality both to ourselves and to those with whom we are in contact. We achieve this by the things we do, what we wear, where we live, the things we say and how we say them, as well as in our art, music and literature. In turn, feedback received from others influences how we see ourselves. If other people consistently label us as untidy, we will eventually incorporate the idea of untidiness into our own self-perception. We have to establish new relationships with people as well as maintain old ones and we have to declare those relationships to others. We have to explore ourselves and our environment in order to learn and control our environment either directly by our own behaviour, or indirectly through other people. We can either shut a window or ask someone else to do it for us. Just how the request is made will determine whether or not the window is eventually closed. To do all these things we have to be able to receive information and to pass information on to others.

HOW DO WE COMMUNICATE?

We are all experts in communicating and normally do not consciously analyse what is involved. Often it is not until something goes wrong and someone breaks one of the many unwritten rules of communication that we focus on our behaviour and that of others. Certainly the ways in which we communicate are subtle and complex but they can be observed and identified. We each have an inherent and extensive knowledge of how communication works which, once it is brought to our conscious attention, can be fitted into a framework. It is helpful to break the complex act of communicating into the following groups of component behaviours.

Group 1

    speaking
    listening
    writing
    reading

These behaviours involve the use of words in some form to convey meaning. Broadly speaking they tend to yield the factual content of a message.

Group 2

    intonation
    volume
    pitch level
    voice quality
    rate of speech
    stress

These behaviours do use voice and although they themselves are not words, they are usually dependent on words. It is not possible to have a rate of speech without speaking, but an intonation pattern can be superimposed onto sounds other than words.

Group 3

space
gaze
posture
facial expression
gesture
touch
dress

This group consists of non-verbal behaviours whose function varies. They can stand in place of words and carry a specific meaning as in shaking the head, clenching the fist or shrugging the shoulders. They can also supplement a verbal message as in nodding the head and saying 'yes', or crooking a finger and saying 'Come here'. Non-verbal messages tell us about the social and emotional content of an exchange. What do the participants feel about each other? Do they like each other? Are they agreeing or disagreeing? How well do they know each other? Are they equals or is there some status difference between them?

Group 4

yawning
laughing
sighing
coughing
'er'
'umm'
'ahh'

These behaviours are used in a variety of ways. They do involve the use of voice but not words. They are more likely to contribute to the social and emotional content of a message.

For the present purpose we shall call the behaviours listed in group 1 verbal behaviour, and place groups 2, 3 and 4 together for consideration as non-verbal behaviour.

SPEECH AND LANGUAGE

We will begin by examining the verbal behaviours listed in group 1. Although the terms speech and language are often used interchangeably they are not synonymous and we need to distinguish between them. Language refers to our ability to manipulate symbols. A symbol is something that stands in place of something else, whether an object such as a table, or a concept such as 'height' or 'yesterday'.

The picture in Fig. 1.1 stands in place of the real thing, as do the printed marks BOOK, the sound 'book' and the gesture shown in picture form in Fig. 1.2. Not only are we able to link symbols with the thing they represent but also with each other and hence we know that all the symbols in Fig. 1.3 are inter-related.

The symbols used most frequently are words although these do not always have to be spoken aloud. We think in words and it is

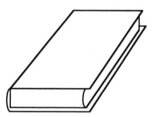

Fig. 1.1 The picture symbol stands in place of the real object.

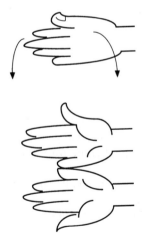

Fig. 1.2 The gesture represented here stands in place of the real object.

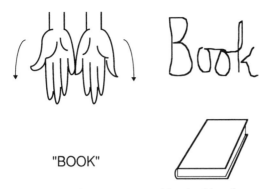

"BOOK"

Fig. 1.3 All these symbols are connected by the idea they represent.

very difficult to keep them out of our thoughts. Spend a couple of minutes thinking about anything at all but trying to keep words away. If a word does come into your head attempt to push it back. This will be difficult if not impossible to do, for whilst we can think visually to some extent, we largely depend on verbal symbols to structure our thoughts and ideas. The term 'language' refers to this ability to manipulate symbols whether they are spoken words, written words, pictures or gestures.

Different cultures use different symbol systems or languages, most of which are based on words. However, it is possible to have picture and gesture languages as in the hieroglyphics of ancient civilizations and the sign systems used by deaf people, some of which can be classified as languages in their own right.

Language expression and comprehension

Communication involves the transfer of symbols from the mind of one person to that of another and is accomplished by speaking, writing, drawing or using gestures. To complete the process it is also necessary to receive and interpret those symbols that are produced for us by other people. Hence language is said to have an expressive function (the production of symbols) and a receptive function (the understanding of symbols). The latter is often called comprehension and includes understanding of the spoken word, written word, pictures and gestures.

Anatomically the traditional understanding is that the symbolic activity of language is organized in the temporo-parietal region of the left cerebral hemisphere and that, unlike many other functions,

5

it is not bilaterally represented in the brain. However language is an extraordinarily complex phenomenon and it is now seen as simplistic to say that its organization is restricted to one particular area. Normal functioning is dependent on many inter-related and intact cognitive skills and therefore involves many different areas of the brain. The importance of the right cerebral hemisphere in the processing of language is currently receiving attention. For some time it has been acknowledged that when damage to the language areas of the left hemisphere occurs in children before the time linked with prime language acquisition, the right hemisphere can assume some language function in its place. Its potential for doing this declines beyond that point. In a normal person the right hemisphere is generally considered to be involved in higher language functions. In *The Right Hemisphere Language Battery* (1989), Bryan identifies the key relevant skill areas:

1. Metaphor
Our day-to-day language is liberally scattered with figures of speech which have to be interpreted non-literally in order to be understood, e.g. a heavy heart, green fingers, a soft option. Right brain-damaged individuals find it hard to deal with the non-literal aspects of language.

2. Comprehension of inferred meaning
Much of our understanding requires us to move a step further than the presented material, i.e. to infer certain meanings from the information already given, for example, 'She was walking around town with a heavy coat on' (in other words we assume it is winter).

3. Humour
Jokes, sarcasm and humour generally rely heavily on metaphor and inferred meaning for their effect. Right brain-damaged people find it hard to appreciate verbal humour.

4. Prosody
This refers to features such as rhythm, stress and intonation patterns which influence the meaning of an utterance. For example, if we consider stress (how much emphasis is placed on a syllable), it can be seen that the meaning of the following sentence varies slightly depending on which word is stressed:

I want to go to town tomorrow.
I *want* to go to town tomorrow.
I want to *go* to town tomorrow.
I want to go to *town* tomorrow.
I want to go to town *tomorrow*.

5.   Discourse analysis
The right hemisphere is needed to achieve a synthesis of all the skills needed to understand the overall meaning of any communication and in order to produce normal language.

THE PRODUCTION OF SPEECH

Speech refers to the production of a particular set of symbols, namely spoken words. It depends on the inter-dependent functioning of the following:

Respiration	abdominal muscles and diaphragm, intercostal muscles.
Phonation	laryngeal muscles, vocal cords.
Articulation	middle, anterior and posterior tongue muscles; facial muscles, especially those for lip-rounding, retracting, opening and closing; palatopharyngeal muscles; mandible and related muscles; pharyngeal muscles.

Respiration

Breathing provides an energy source for speech in the form of a moving airstream. This can be likened to the petrol supply in a car where an ample supply must be fed through at a controlled rate. A good breath capacity maintains adequate volume and enables speech to be phrased appropriately. Normally speech occurs only on the expiratory phase of the breathing cycle on an egressive airstream (although it is possible to phonate whilst breathing in). More control is needed in breathing for speech than in quiet respiration, the expiratory phase of the cycle being longer than it is for quiet breathing. During speaking episodes the descent of the rib cage is controlled by the intercostal muscles. This is in contrast to quiet respiration where descent of the rib

7

cage is brought about by the elastic recoil of the lungs. Good control of expiration and inspiration ensures that stress and intonation patterns are not disturbed.

Phonation

Sound is produced in the larynx which is a cartilaginous tube at the top of the trachea. The larynx changes its position in the neck on swallowing and during alterations in vocal pitch. Placing the fingers lightly over the larynx during a swallow enables the larynx to be felt moving upwards and then down again before returning to a rest position. Similar changes can be felt or observed while humming up or down a scale. The vocal cords (sometimes called vocal folds) are two sheets of muscle stretched across the larynx each of which is attached anteriorly to a small triangular cartilage, the arytenoid cartilage. During quiet respiration the cords are abducted but on phonation they are adducted by the arytenoids (Fig. 1.4a and b).

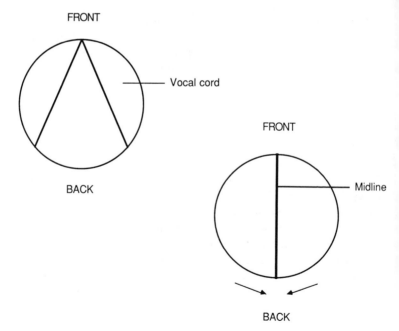

Fig. 1.4 (a) Vocal cord abduction during respiration; (b) vocal cord adduction during phonation.

8

On adduction the edges of the cords meet and as air is forced upwards from the lungs, the pressure in the vocal tract below the cords increases until they are blown apart, releasing a puff of air into the vocal tract immediately above. Consequently the pressure below the cords drops and they are sucked back together again (the Bernouilli effect). The cycle is repeated many times each second, causing the column of air above the cords to vibrate. This vibration is perceived as sound. The cords move too rapidly for the vibration to be seen with the naked eye, but individual cycles of opening and closing can be viewed using a flexible fibre-optic rhinolaryngoscope (FFRL) linked to a stroboscope (Chapter 6) or alternatively they can be displayed on a laryngograph.

The noise made at the level of the larynx is thin and reedy but it is amplified as a result of the resonance set up in the rest of the vocal tract and in the bony cavities or sinuses of the skull. The final quality of the sound depends on the unique anatomy and muscle tone of an individual's vocal tract. This means that every voice is different, in face voices are so distinctive that it is usually possible to identify someone by the sound of their voice alone.

For good voice we need to maintain an adequate volume and to have fine control over the laryngeal muscles in order to coordinate breathing and phonation and to bring about the subtle changes in cord tension necessary for pitch change and intonation. We can change the overall pitch of our voice by increasing the frequency of cord vibration and the position of the larynx in the neck. Intonation refers to the small alterations in pitch that continuously occur from syllable to syllable when speaking.

Articulation

Precise consonant and vowel formation involves contact or near contact (approximation) between two articulators. The active or moveable articulators are the lips, tongue, soft palate and lower jaw. The passive or immovable articulators are the upper jaw, hard palate and upper teeth. Normal articulation requires very rapid and accurate movements of the articulators in order to transfer precisely from one sound to another, particularly where clusters or groups of consonants are concerned. Some clusters found in English are:

sp	as in	speech
kr	as in	cream
pl	as in	plane
str	as in	string
kspl	as in	explore

NON-VERBAL BEHAVIOUR

In order to make a starting point we will consider some of the important non-verbal behaviours in group 3 individually but it will soon become apparent that even within this group they are inter-related and that in our normal interactions we simultaneously analyse and cross-reference many different component signals from all the groups.

Space

The study of spacing, or where we physically place ourselves with respect to other people, is called proxemics. We all feel comfortable with different amounts of physical space between ourselves and another person depending on the situation. The better we know someone the less we need to maintain space between us and them, so as we become more familiar with a person we hold conversations at progressively smaller distances, hence we stand closer to friends than to strangers.

The type of interaction and with whom it takes place will determine how comfortable we are at any given distance. It is easy to test out personal space. Stand still and ask a friend to move slowly towards you one step at a time. At each step consider whether to give permission for the friend to come closer or not. Make sure you ask them to take smaller steps as the distance between you decreases. You will know when the closest comfortable distance has been reached because there will be an impulse to lean away or to step back. Try to pay attention to which part of your body registers the discomfort (it may be a generalized feeling that you cannot localize). Repeat the experiment with someone taller or smaller, with someone of the opposite sex and when you are sitting on a chair. Experiment with space at social gatherings by moving closer to one particular person. They will probably adjust their spacing in some way without realizing they are responding to you.

Spacing is an effective indicator of the status and power that is operating in a relationship. Powerful people are given, or take, more space. A hospital consultant will have an office of his own, whereas a cleaner in the same building will be lucky to get a locker in the basement. In some circumstances space is divided on a first come, first served basis. Open spaces such as a beach, a picnic area or a restaurant are filled systematically with the first arrivals spreading over large areas and the late-comers then having to fill in the spaces left between those who have already established their territory.

Closing off another person's space by purposely standing or sitting too near or leaning more than halfway across a desk will usually be perceived as threatening behaviour, unless something has been done or said to excuse and acknowledge the act. This is why we mutter something such as 'Excuse me' when reaching across someone.

Vertical space is just as important as horizontal space. Important people are placed 'higher up' (and it is worth noting how many of our common idioms reflect their origin in non-verbal behaviour) on thrones, a dais or a platform. We make ourselves lower as a sign of respect by bowing, curtseying or prostrating ourselves. It is harder to feel dominant when another person is taller than ourselves.

Gaze

To meet another person's gaze is a social act which has many functions. When we look at someone we gather information about them from their appearance and their behaviour. Two people who make eye-contact (mutual gaze) are signalling that they wish to start an interaction. A listener indicates an interest in what is being said and a liking for the other speaker by frequent eye-contacts of short duration. Our pupils dilate when we look at someone we like and thus we tend to like people who have large pupils.

In conversations we take turns to speak and a speaker will use eye-contact to show the listener he wishes to relinquish a speaking turn. He will usually start to make longer and longer glances at the listener just before the end of a period of speaking to signal

11

that the listener can take over if he wishes. Listeners generally look at speakers more than speakers look at listeners unless the speaker is of higher status. Staring at a speaker too much will make it harder for him to plan the next bit of his speaking and therefore increase his speech errors. For this reason when we are speaking and searching for a word or planning what to say next, we avert our gaze.

Conversely, a listener will indicate that he wants to interrupt by trying to establish eye-contact with the speaker, changing posture, maybe sitting forward in the chair, and taking an audible inward breath. Having prepared the ground in this way he hopes that when he begins to speak the other will back down. Two people talking at the same time are not communicating so usually someone stops. They may negotiate who is to carry on both verbally and non-verbally – 'After you', 'No you', etc. If the listener repeatedly fails to get in on a turn he will have to take stronger measures and will start the challenge by speaking slightly louder and quicker than he would normally.

On the other hand if a listener does not want a turn he will avoid eye-contact. At school we were all familiar with staring at our books when the class was asked a question. In the same way asking a group for volunteers will usually lead to a sudden interest in the floor! Eye-contact also indicates status. The more dominant person is allowed to make more direct eye-contact and maintain it for longer. Eye-contact maintained for longer than our own cultural code allows in a specific situation is perceived as bold or threatening.

There is an inverse relationship between eye-contact and spacing so that for a constant relationship the closer you are physically to a person, the less you will look at him. However we allow ourselves more eye-contact with people we know better. The extreme of this is demonstrated by lovers who usually indulge in a lot of eye-contact at close physical distances. When testing our your personal space with another person notice what happens to your eye-contact as you approach them. It is likely to decrease except for occasional glances to check out possible reactions. At these points you will be inclined to smile, a way of acknowledging that the situation which could be potentially threatening is in fact alright.

Posture

Posture indicates the emotional state of a person but it also gives information about the social relationship between two or more people. Within a group people unconsciously use posture to define the limits of that group and to restrict access to it. If the group is free standing then its members will tend to form a circle.

Orientation

This is the angle two people adopt towards each other. Different orientations inhibit or facilitate eye-contact and thus give clues about the nature of the exchange. For competitive interactions such as interviewing, examining or arguing, people sit opposite each other (facing), whereas for cooperative interactions they tend to sit corner to corner or side by side (parallel) (Argyle, 1983).

If seating arrangements limit the orientation such that people are unable to signal with their whole body, they will still signal orientation by the position of their head and extremities. If a group is sitting in a line, the two end members will turn in and close off the group by extending an arm or leg across the free space. Orientation is often split so that no members of the group are excluded and so the trunk, head and arms can be turned towards one person, while the legs and feet are turned towards another. Thus everyone in the group is included as facing or parallel with some other member.

Congruence

This refers to the degree of similarity between the postures of two people and is reflected by the adoption of identical positions or those that are mirror images, such as having opposite legs crossed. It is more likely to occur between people who like each other and it indicates some degree of identification with the other person. In groups with up to six members, when one person shifts and changes position the others will shortly follow suit and so congruence is maintained. Congruence is less likely to occur when there is a difference in status. Even when two parties are disagreeing, continued congruence of part of the body indicates the continuance of the relationship despite the disagreement. This signalling of relationships is largely unconscious. Imagine you are at a party, it has been a long day and you are tired, your feet ache and you are desperate to sit down. At one end of the room is a small two-seater sofa and a person you have never seen before is seated at one end. Finally you simply have to rest and sit down on the vacant end of the sofa. How do you sit? How do you orientate your legs and what do you do with your arms? You will probably sit close to the end of the sofa and as far as possible from the stranger, thus obeying the spacing rules. You may also have your legs crossed away from the stranger and are likely to lean your outer arm on that of the sofa. You may perch on the edge of the seat. What you are doing is signalling both to the stranger and to the rest of the room, that you do not know and have no relationship with the person next to you. These signals will be more overt if it is someone of the opposite sex. Conversely the limits of available space may mean it is impossible to maintain a comfortable distance with the stranger however you position yourself. In this situation if you cannot change the spacing, you may have to change the relationship and will make eye-contact and some superficial conversation so that the person is no longer a complete stranger. If the same scenario is changed slightly such that there are two people already sitting on a three-seater sofa and your only option is to sit in the middle, then you are likely to hold your arms close to your body and keep your legs uncrossed. You will also be more inclined to perch on the edge of the seat.

Generally, when posture is used to indicate status, the more powerful a person is, the more they can afford to use a relaxed posture in front of others.

Facial expression

Some basic facial expressions such as those for happiness (smiling), grief (frowning, crying) and anger (teeth baring, snarling, sneering) are signals that are common across cultures and to some animals as well (Morris, 1981). They can be considered as a particular type of gesture (see below). Many facial expressions are under our conscious control, they have specific names and we can produce them at will. These include smiling, frowning and pouting. Others, like changes in forehead skin tension or more subtle variations in lip position, are not so specific or easily labelled. We continuously monitor facial expressions to supply us with feedback during conversations.

Gesture

A gesture gives information to an onlooker and can take the form of an intentional signal, like waving, or an unintentional one. We can describe different categories of gestures:

1. Some gestures are independent of speech. They replace words and have a strong communicative import. They are sent and received quite consciously, e.g. nodding, waving, thumbs up and down, and beckoning. A particular application of this type of gesture is found in formal sign languages and systems.

2. Some facial expressions and limb movements are used to supplement speech. The command 'Come here' is often used with a beckoning movement. The expression of disgust 'Ugh' is nearly always used with a corresponding physical expression of disgust such as wrinkling the nose. Try saying 'Ugh' with the same amount of feeling but without the accompanying nose wrinkle. It can be done but it feels odd. We often add emphasis to our words by gesturing. What sort of gestures might accompany the words 'I DON'T want to go!' or 'The point I'm TRYING to make is . . .'?

3. We obtain feedback in conversations by watching the other person's gestures. These may include shrugs, nods, shaking the head, tapping fingers, raising eyebrows, fidgeting with fingers and rubbing hands together. These gestures are predominantly involuntary.

4. Gestures are used to regulate conversations. In this way they enable us to negotiate who talks when and for how long. They help us to attract attention, to interrupt and to terminate a conversation satisfactorily. The use of gestures in this way has been extensively studied and varying theories have been advanced. It has been suggested that certain gestures, mainly small eye and head movements, mark our spoken phrases, sentences and paragraphs in much the same way as written language is punctuated by commas and full stops.

Gestures are powerful indicators of power and status in a relationship. They are culturally determined in the same way as other aspects of non-verbal behaviour. The Western gesture of touching the tips of the thumb and index finger to form a circle in Britain and America signals OK, in France zero, in Japan money and in Tunisia 'I'll kill you'! If you ask a shepherd in Afghanistan whether you are on the right road an upward lift of the head indicates 'yes', whereas if you want to flag down a taxi in Northern Nigeria you must extend your arm forwards and downwards with the palm facing down and wave your hand at the ground.

Touch

Touch as a means of communication has largely been suppressed in most Western cultures and tends to be either formalized as in hand-shaking or reserved for intimate relationship. Otherwise if we accidentally touch part of another person's body with our own we apologize. Even the innocent person is likely to mutter an apology and so there is a joint acknowledgement of the incident.

Some forms of touching are allowed because they are contained within the boundaries of a specific situation, such as massage, nursing care, physiotherapy, beauty therapy, hair dressing, dentistry or a game of rugby.

Touch is powerful and should be used with respect for the other person. In a clinical setting it should be acceptable to the client as well as to the person offering the contact. It is important to remember that our own degree of comfort or discomfort with touch may not be shared by the client.

Dress

Clothes make us comfortable by keeping us warm or cool and they protect us. They enable us to conceal parts of our body and to switch off certain body signals, especially the sexual ones. The rules of modesty vary from culture to culture both geographically and historically so that the Victorian habit of even covering the legs of furniture seems remarkable to us today.

Our dress allows us to identify ourselves with a particular social category and this is the oldest known use of clothing (Morris, 1981). We simultaneously signal which group we belong to or wish to belong to and those groups we do or do not wish to be seen as belonging to. Uniforms especially act in this way and although not all uniforms are formal, they are strong markers of status. In

British hospitals consultants usually wear smart dark suits as an unofficial uniform while their more junior colleagues wear white coats. Uniforms in hospitals serve many purposes including hygiene, protection and identification, but do uniforms in this context hinder or facilitate communication?

Rules about what we wear depend on the occasion and we expend much time, effort and money in getting it right. When we fail, for example by going to a party dressed more formally than any one else, we feel extremely uncomfortable. If we are unsure about the nature of a specific social event we tend to play safe and wear something non-committal that we hope will be acceptable across a range of eventualities.

Clothes influence how we feel about ourselves and therefore how we project ourselves to other people. When I first qualified as a therapist I always wore my white coat to see clients. It made me feel more confident and I hoped it would make me appear competent. As I became more sure of myself I still wore a coat on the wards because I needed to convince other staff that I knew what I was doing, but I no longer wore it to see out-patients (although when I anticipated a 'difficult' client I would slip it on again). Later still there seemed no reason even to wear the coat on the wards as it had become a barrier that hindered my interaction with the clients and I then stopped wearing it altogether.

Sometimes clothes are used consciously to control an interaction or to give a particular impression, hence most of us dress smartly for an interview. In the same way patients who come to see a doctor may dress to hide their distress, depression or illness.

Removing a patient's clothes removes many personal signals. The custom of undressing a person before the doctor arrives may save time but it also makes it easier for the doctor to regard the patient as just another body in the daily routine. Certainly the absence of clothes helps to remove any status the person may have. It is very hard to be assertive when you are practically naked and the other person is fully dressed. The converse of this effect is sometimes used in assertiveness training as a strategy to enable people to feel more confident and act more assertively with a particular individual. Here the person who feels dominated is asked to visualize their protagonist in underwear, or in some other dress that makes them less threatening, such as old gardening clothes.

CULTURAL VARIATION

It is important to remember that except for some basic facial expressions, all non-verbal behaviours are culturally determined. Thus the meaning of the same piece of behaviour differs from one culture to another (Fig. 1.1). We learn these cultural specific behaviours by watching other people. Both individual gestures and clusters of gestures have different meanings and are to be interpreted differently according to culture and context. The lowered head and averted gaze of an Asian woman is a mark of respect, whereas in the west she might be thought sad, uncooperative, sulky or shy. Such differences in non-verbal codes can make it harder to form very close friendships with people from different cultures.

Personal space varies a great deal from culture to culture, the concept itself seeming to be almost non-existent in some places and hallowed in others. This may depend on the amount of personal space experienced as a child. If you grow up living in the same room as ten other people, personal space will mean something very different from growing up in a house where you have your own bedroom. An English lecturer in northern Nigeria was discomfitted by the way his students leaned right across his desk in conversation or moved uninvited round to his side, standing close to look over the work. In a western culture this could indicate disrespect or a challenge to authority, yet these students were not intending any disrespect as their other behaviours, such as backing out the door and lowering their heads, indicated deference.

Our rules concerning the use of touch are also culturally based and so some groups are happier with physical contact than others. Touching occurs more between Arabs, Latin Americans and South Europeans than between North Europeans, North Americans or Asians. Both same sex and cross sex touching varies. In northern Nigeria it is common to see men holding hands while walking and talking and women too will touch each other in this way. However the idea of opposite sex friends touching in public is quite preposterous, even if they are man and wife.

NON-VERBAL SIGNALS IN CONTEXT

Playing detective by observing non-verbal behaviour is a fascinating pastime but it is easy to be misled. No one piece of behaviour means any one thing. It is unwise simply to say that when a man strokes his chin he is making a decision (Pease, 1981). We have to analyse his total behaviour and use this to arrive at a viable conclusion.

When people are bored in a lecture or meeting they are well aware it is not acceptable to say aloud 'This is boring'. However they do have their own well-being to consider and so they begin to give the speaker messages that all is not well. These messages will not be intrusive and will not interrupt the speaker's flow. Perhaps people begin to shuffle and change their posture more frequently. They may fiddle with their fingers, hair or a piece of clothing. They may glance at a watch and their eyes will wander away from the speaker for longer and longer periods.

If the speaker is competent he will notice these cues and introduce a break or do something to regain the group's interest. If he is either not aware of the messages or incapable of changing the situation the audience will be forced to deliver more and more overt messages. Hence their shuffling will become more frequent, there will be audible sighs, eye-contact with diminish still further and yawns will creep in despite attempts to stifle them. The most overt signal the audience could give would be to get up and leave but this is very confrontational and most people would not feel able to do this except as an extreme measure.

However, the speaker needs to be aware of possible explanations for the behaviour other than boredom. He needs to consider whether the seats are comfortable and whether the audience has been sitting in them for a long time. Are some listeners tired and is the room too hot or too cold? The physical, social and emotional context of a situation must be taken into account before arriving at any conclusions.

SPLIT MESSAGES

We feel most comfortable when the non-verbal messages complement and agree with the verbal ones, but they often do not. When they disagree it is an indication of the power of non-verbal signals that we automatically accept the non-verbal one as being correct. A contradictory non-verbal message can not only dilute a verbal message but can completely reverse its meaning. To demonstrate this we really need to hear a spoken message but some parallels can be presented on the page:

I'm NOT angry!'

What is the real message of this speaker? We tend to become more aware of non-verbal behaviours when we are sending or receiving mixed messages. Convincing someone that you are full of the joys of spring when in fact you are really feeling exhausted and depressed takes a lot of effort. You would be very conscious of that effort and unlikely to be convincing. We become aware of the non-verbal system when we or someone else breaks our cultural code. Foreigners break our rules simply because their own are different. Children regularly do because they have not yet learned them and although we are prepared to accept this, they are not permitted to act in this way as they eventually have to learn the correct behaviours. Such errors tend to elicit the following sorts of responses from accompanying adults:

'Don't stare, it's rude.'
'Don't interrupt when I'm talking.'
'Take your hand away from your mouth.'
'Sit still.'
'Look at me when I'm talking.'
'Don't fidget.'

Mentally handicapped people often break the unwritten rules of non-verbal behaviour. They will stand too close, hug, kiss and touch when it is not appropriate for any other adult to do so. This is one of the reasons why it is hard for some people to feel comfortable in the presence of the mentally handicapped.

CAN WE NOT COMMUNICATE?

Consider this question in the light of what has been discussed so far. Imagine a person who is trying hard not to communicate anything at all. How and where would they sit? What facial expression might they have? What would their eye-contact be like? Keep the scene in your mind's eye for a few seconds. Do you get any 'feel' about the person at all? If you do then they must be communicating something. The messages may be along the lines of 'I'm fed up', 'I'm depressed', 'I'm sulking' or 'I don't want to talk', all of which are far from indicating an absence of communication. On the contrary they are strong messages.

If you were instructed to go to work tomorrow with an observer and to go about your normal duties without communicating with anyone in any way whatsoever, what sort of things would you be able to do? The answer is likely to be nothing. Your behaviour will continuously leak signals to the observer. It is impossible not to behave and therefore impossible not to communicate.

This concept has great significance when it comes to considering people who have communication disorders. If we as human beings are communicating all the time and that communication is impaired for some reason, then our functioning is impaired all the time. Thus having a communication disorder is about more than not being able to ask for a cup of tea or not being able to chat about what happened yesterday. Rather it is a diminishing of performance that extends through every waking moment of a person's life.

CLASSIFICATION OF COMMUNICATION DISORDERS

Because of their diverse nature, communication disorders are difficult to classify but the following systems are often used (Crystal, 1980).

Classification by symptom

This is perhaps the most widely used system.

1. Disorders of language (e.g. developmental language disorders, dysphasia, schizophrenic language, the language of dementia).
2. Disorders of voluntary movement (e.g. dyspraxia).
3. Disorders of articulation (e.g. dysarthria, cleft palate).
4. Disorders of voice (e.g. dysphonia, pitch disorders).
5. Disorders of fluency (e.g. stammering).
6. Disorders of hearing.

It is important to remember that more than one symptom of impaired communication may be present at the same time and thus after a stroke any one person may demonstrate some degree of dysphasia (language), dyspraxia (voluntary movement) and dysarthria (articulation).

Classification by time of onset

Communication disorders can be either congenital, or developmental or they may be acquired at some point after the normal acquisition of skills has taken place, as a result of accident or illness. In daily use the term developmental disorder is more likely to refer to a child and an acquired disorder to an adult. Obviously children can acquire disorders as a result of trauma or disease and the effects of a developmental disorder may persist into adulthood.

Classification by degree

Symptoms are described as being mild, moderate or severe, thus someone may have a severe or a mild dysarthria.

Classification by aetiology

Not all communication disorders have a physical cause, some are psychological in origin. It is possible to have a dysphonia of organic aetiology but some dysphonias are psychogenic. There is often considerable interplay between organic and non-organic factors. Some symptoms, like dysfluency, may have several possible aetiologies.

THE SIZE OF THE PROBLEM

For a long time it has been difficult to gain any clear idea as to how many communication disordered people there are. To some extent this is because they do not form a homogeneous group and communication disorders occur across a wide variety of medical specialities. In 1986 Enderby and Philipp published estimates for the UK of the number of people with communication problems, grouped in different medical categories. They concluded that '. . . 2.3 million people in the UK have some sort of speech or language disorder. Of these 800,000 have a severe communication disorder (i.e. have difficulty making themselves understood by anyone other than their immediate family), and 1.5 million have a moderate communication disorder (i.e. a speech and language deficit which is noticeable to the lay person but who may nevertheless remain intelligible).' The authors point out that their figures do not include data on autism, mutism, stammering, psychological speech loss, familiar dystonias and psychiatric speech disturbances. As these additional areas contribute significantly to the caseload carried by many communication therapy clinics, it can be assumed that, if anything, the size of the communication disordered population in the UK is well in excess of the figures quoted above.

WHOSE RESPONSIBILITY?

Communication disorder is an umbrella term covering a wide range of impairments that traditionally have poor status both in the medical and social services. Unfortunately public awareness of both the existence and nature of communication disorders is less advanced than for many other handicaps that are more easily understood. All too often professionals not directly involved in the field are ill-equipped to manage such clients, largely as a result of inadequate or non-existent training. Communication disorders are frequently dealt with, if at all, in an ad hoc fashion on many professional undergraduate courses such as medicine and nursing. This is despite the fact that many of these students will spend a large part of their professional lives dealing with patients who have impaired communication of one sort or another.

This lack of preparation makes it hard for those professionals who later come into contact with communication disordered people to appreciate the physical, psychological and social impact of a communication deficit. As a consequence, when there is a multiple disability such as brain damage following a stroke or head injury, the communication deficit is regarded as being the least distressing and disabling symptom. This could hardly be further from the truth. The social and psychological implications will be discussed more fully in Chapter 9, but we have already

2

Talking to people with communication disorders

LANGUAGE STYLES

We are familiar with the idea of different styles of written language being employed in different circumstances. Our own experience will determine how well we are able to interpret each one. Even if we do not know exactly what is meant we can at least identify the style and hence make some guess at the context. Usually we know which style to use in which context or, conversely, we can guess the context from the style. Look at this passage.

MEMORANDUM OF AGREEMENT made this 8th day of November 1989 between Eleanor Withington (hereinafter called 'the AUTHOR' which expression shall, where the context admits, include the AUTHOR's executors, administrators and assigns) of the one part and Parker and Thom on behalf of the Scientific, Technical and Medical Publishing Division of Le Boutillier, Parker and Thom (UK) LTD of 7 Cotton Rd., London, and of 26 East 42nd Street, New York, USA (hereinafter called 'the PUBLISHERS' assigns or successors in business as the case may be) of the other part. WHEREAS the AUTHOR is writing, compiling or editing a literary work (hereinafter referred to as 'the work') at present entitled: VOCAL CORD PATHOLOGY consisting of between 160 and 180 printed pages calculated at 500 words per page but with due allowance for illustrations and/or formulae, now it is mutually agreed between the parties hereto as follows:

Here we have what is actually quite a restrained piece of legalese in which the publishers of the book are merely saying 'This is a contract'. Different language styles allow varying degrees of formality and precision. Notice how the terms themselves are defined, even though words like 'author' and 'publisher' are well-known words. Some of the vocabulary is archaic, where else would you find words like 'hereinafter' and 'hereto'? The sentences are long and rambling with many clauses inserted into them. It takes some concentration to remember what topic the sentence originally started on. Such a prose style hardly makes for gripping reading but achieves a purpose, which is to cover as many loose ends as possible and avoid any ambiguity of meaning, that is if you can follow it. A lawyer trained in legalese may understand his documents; the rest of us usually struggle to make sense of them, although when confronted with one we have no doubt that it is a legal document. We recognize the style.

Scientific research articles provide another example of language which intends to be absolutely precise in its meaning but achieves this in a different manner from 'legalese'. Most scientific disciplines develop a specific vocabulary which may include words not used in everyday speech and invented specially, or words which sound familiar but are used in a different way. Each discipline acquires its own 'buzz' phrases. Even if you belong to one scientific discipline and understand its vocabulary, that does not necessarily mean you have any facility with the written language of a different discipline. I can understand medical languages but would be baffled if I tried to read a piece on computer science. Consider this statement.

$$\sum_{n=1}^{\infty} \frac{1}{n^2} = \frac{\pi^2}{6}$$

Yes, it is maths but that is as far as I can get, although I do recognize some vocabulary such as 'pi squared' and 'infinity'. Sometimes mathematical statements use words and we might expect these to be a bit easier for non-mathematicians to grasp. Look at Cauchy's Theorem.

If $f(z)$ is analytic in the region Ω, which is simply connected, and α is a closed curve in Ω, then

$$\int_\alpha f(z)dz = 0$$

Any the wiser? Even though we know the vocabulary, the words and phrases are obviously being used in a very different way. In one sense I can understand the phrase 'and is simply connected' but in the theorem this phrase is apparently being used to mean something extra. The mathematical system almost eradicates the ambiguity of verbal languages mainly by using different symbols, the meaning of which are logically defined. Any academic discipline strives to make its language clear of ambiguities and yet sometimes ambiguity is necessary. Poetic styles, whether in poetry or prose, rely on a more open use of language where the meaning isn't so defined for their power and effect. In this way a writer can invoke layers of meaning simultaneously so that one piece can work at several levels. In its own way poetic language can be just as difficult to 'understand' as scientific forms of expression. Our day-to-day written language styles fluctuate somewhere between these two extremes.

So it is in spoken language. We not only adapt our non-verbal behaviour to match the situation and the person we are speaking to, we also adapt our language. On overhearing a conversation between two strangers, it is possible to make a good guess as to whether they are employer and employee, two friends, colleagues, strangers, or lovers, based on the way they speak to each other. Similarly, different speech styles are appropriate for a classroom, a courtroom, a party, an interview, or a debate. Language is modified to make it simpler when we perceive our listener to be linguistically or cognitively less competent than ourselves. Thus simplified styles are used with foreigners, children, old people, animals, babies and people with communication disorders.

As infants we hear others address us in the linguistic style of baby talk. Even without being linguists there is something about the next passage that means we know the story is being told to a child rather than an adult.

When Tess and Michael arrived at the seaside they were very excited. They took off their shoes and socks and ran as fast as they could to the sea. Oh it was cold! The waves splashed and gurgled over their feet. The water foamed on the sand and dragged at their toes. They laughed and shouted at each other, delighted to be on holiday at last.

27

In the same way we can tell the next passage is intended for a younger child.

> Sammy the snail squiggled and wriggled. He huffed and puffed and a tear trickled down his grey cheek. 'What's the matter?' asked Mark the mouse. 'I've lost my house', sobbed Sammy. 'Lost your house?' 'Yes, lost my house.' 'Oh dear,' muttered Mark. He cleaned a whisker while he thought about things. 'Oh dear, oh dear, oh dear,' he said, 'What a terrible thing.'

How do we know? To some extent the content gives us clues but there are other markers that we unconsciously pick up on. Baby talk has been studied extensively by linguists and it is possible to analyse exactly how people adapt their language when they talk to babies or young children. Specific features of speech to children include:

1. simpler linguistic forms;
2. more redundant language ie. lots of repetitions;
3. shorter utterances;
4. a higher proportion of questions;
5. a higher proportion of commands;
6. a slower rate of speech.

There is also a tendency to use a greater volume, more exaggerated intonation patterns and exaggerated facial expressions.

One problem with this style of language is that it tends to be generalized to inappropriate situations and thus baby talk is frequently used for speaking to old people and patients in hospital. When an elderly person accuses a nurse of treating her like a child, it is likely to be the nurse's style of communication that is the culprit.

Most of us are guilty of using baby talk inappropriately in this way at some time or other although we are unlikely to be aware of doing it. Baby talk is easy to hear. Listen for it from well-meaning staff in hospital lifts, waiting-rooms and clinics. You may well hear something along the following lines.

> Right, Mr Blake, let's have you in this chair now shall we? Can you manage? Sure? Take it easy. No need to rush. Slowly. Nearly there. OK.? Now then, what would you like

for supper? Fish? A nice casserole? Sausages? Yes? You sure? Right, sausages it is. Now shall we see what's on the news? Oh and I'll get you some water before I go. There. Don't forget to drink it will you? I'll be off then. Are you going to drink it for me now? Good. Give me the cup. Good. Ring if you want anything, won't you?.

How many elements of baby talk can you identify in the above passage? If you visualize yourself sitting in place of Mr Blake during this exchange, it will serve to highlight the language as inappropriate.

Clients with communication disorders are usually spoken to as if they were either children or stupid. Unfortunately the use of baby talk only exacerbates the communication problem. When there is a comprehension problem, it is necessary to modify language in some way to maximize the client's understanding but baby talk rarely improves understanding. The client would benefit more from being spoken to in one of the modified but appropriate adult language styles described later.

VARIABILITY OF COMMUNICATIVE ABILITY

Our own ability to communicate is not fixed but depends upon our physical, social and emotional environment. Factors which will exert a direct effect include the following.

Time

Being in a hurry makes it more difficult to express our thoughts clearly.

Physical environment

Distracting background noise such as TV, radio, machinery or other people talking makes it hard to concentrate on speaking. In comfortable surroundings we are able to relax and communicate well. When the physical space is arranged in such a way as to be cosy and intimate, we are more likely to disclose information about ourselves to others than when seated in a large cold room.

Status

When talking to someone of perceived superior or inferior status different rules apply, such as who is allowed to interrupt whom and how often. The superior person will be allowed to interrupt more frequently without causing offence to the inferior one. We are inclined to be more formal and to use more polite language to those we see as superior. It is easiest to communicate well with someone of perceived equal status.

Formality

Situations are often contrived to contain different degrees of formality. The more formal the situation the more overt are the rules that govern communication and the greater the penalty for infringement. For example a committee meeting has an accepted form and the members of that meeting would not normally transgress the accepted code of behaviour.

Emotional state

It is harder to express yourself or to retain information when you are nervous or experiencing some extreme emotion. We even use expressions that reflect this, such as 'I was so cross I was speechless!' The best answer to a question often surfaces on the way home from an interview and it is usually a struggle to remember many of the questions that were asked during it. How often do you replay dialogue in your head after an argument, delivering dazzling repartee that would have floored your opponent had you been able to produce it at the time?

Physical state

Pain or other physical discomfort such as cold may make it harder for us to concentrate and hence communicate to the best of our ability. Tiredness can give rise to a temporary fall in reasoning, sequencing and memory skills, 'I'm too tired to think straight', or even naming problems, 'Oh, what's his name?'. If you have ever had to get out of bed suddenly to speak on the telephone you may have noticed that your speech was slightly slurred.

The influences we have considered here are by no means exhaustive but they do give some idea of the resultant complexity and vulnerability of a process that is dependent on so many interacting factors. Whereabouts a person is performing on their communicative ability continuum at any one time will vary according to the total situation. In general we perform better when relaxed, confident and physically comfortable and less well when tense, anxious and tired or physically unwell. The same applies to someone with a communication disorder. Although he cannot achieve his previous level of ability whatever the environment, his function will still fluctuate across a range depending on the situation (Fig. 2.1).

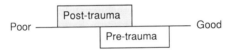

Fig. 2.1 The ranges of communicative ability pre- and post-trauma may overlap.

Doug was a man with a mild communication disorder who had previously worked in a lawyer's office. In the clinic he could have long abstract conversations that to an average listener would have appeared almost normal except for a slight stammer and a tendency to take the long way round when explaining or describing events. However, when given five minutes in front of a doctor in a busy out-patient clinic, Doug could hardly get a word out. He once refused admission for the investigation of persistent headaches because he was only too aware of the traumatic negative effect the ward environment would have on his communication. Here is a transcript of a conversation he had with his therapist about the way other people reacted to his speech.

Therapist: What's the worst thing about having a communication disorder?

Doug: It is being unable to find the words and often saying words that's completely wrong. There's a tendency in my family to know what I mean without telling me 'You are wrong'. I use words which they seem to know what I mean but I get irritated when occasionally I use words like 'Pass me the lights' and it's not referent to lights or anything. Lights seems to come up all the time and it's a bit irritating. I get irritated with not being able to find it.

Therapist: How do people react when they meet you for the first time?

Doug: Some people pretend that they don't see anything wrong with the slowness of my speech. Some seem to say 'Oh, it doesn't seem very much', but others, you could tell from their face, their expressions. They think, 'Oh, I've got one here'. You know. 'He's not quite with it' . . . and again it's a little bit, it puts you off. I tend to back away from talking to complete strangers if I can. Stay in the background.

Therapist: Are people helpful?

Doug: I think most people are not helpful. I think most people are busy. They haven't time to wait for you to find what you want to say. Some people are rude. Even to the degree that their facial expressions . . . [Doug raised his eyes to the ceiling in exasperation] . . . when you are . . . as if you are 'Oh, got a right one here'. Most of the people I've come across haven't the time. That's the main thing.

Therapist: How does that make you feel?

Doug: I feel irritable sometimes. I feel sad. Feel as if I'm slightly different than what, certainly I am different than I was before the stroke, but I'm conscious of it more. That I'm not sort of in with him. I'm a little bit of an oddity more than anything.

Therapist: Would it help if people knew more about the sort of problems you have?

Doug: It probably would but I would like to see how you would make more people aware of the position – problems. People don't want to listen. They've got their own little world that they'd rather not want to meet others, not to know others. I'm sorry.

Therapist: If you could give people some advice as to how to help you, what would it be?

Doug: Be patient. I have occasions when nothing comes out and I think people if they can see someone struggling, to be patient and then that I'm sure would be . . . If they could see someone struggling, to be patient . . . and if I could hope people were patient, and even if they feel as I've said, they sometimes think you're a bit of an oddity, I don't like the . . . [Doug raised his eyes to the ceiling again] . . . if they can keep themselves . . . they don't have to make . . . as if they feel you're mentally ill. Sick. Something like that.

Understanding the significance of the factors that affect communication should place a big responsibility on both the client and those about him to create an environment in which communication can take place at as high a performance level as possible. Unfortunately this doesn't seem to happen automatically, either because people don't realize that physical and social surroundings affect communication or they don't know how to manipulate the environment in such a way as to achieve the best result. It is a sobering thought to realize that what we say and how we say it can not only influence how much a listener understands, but also how much speech they are able to produce. When we have a conversation with someone who has a communication handicap we automatically use some strategies to make things easier. They usually take the form of baby talk. To some extent these strategies are intended to help the other person but they are also used so that we ourselves can negotiate the conversation as comfortably as possible. They usually operate by giving the normal speaker disproportionate control over what is happening. Thus the tendency is for the normal speaker to take on full responsibility for the smooth running of the conversation. This means that on the whole the normal speaker will decide when and where the conversation takes place, what is talked about and how long each topic lasts. He or she will inevitably do most of the talking and use lots of closed questions in an effort to include the other person without making great demands on him. The normal speaker is also the one to decide how and when the conversation finishes.

The balance of the exchange is distorted because normal conversations involve many negotiations where the participants have equal rights even though these rights will vary depending on the speaking situation. The communication impaired person may have unwillingly to surrender his rights and will play little or no active part in the exchange. This is not comfortable for either party and both speakers are likely to feel relieved when the 'conversation' is over. As the normal speaker you may feel forced into behaving in this way by the other person's lack of ability and be unable to see any alternative. However, it is possible to substitute behaviours which leave both parties feeling happier and to reintroduce some balance into the conversation making it less hard work and more rewarding for both. This means that the normal speaker has to acquire some simple skills that can be learned like any other activity. This is not to say that communicating with communication disordered people is easy. It is intrinsically difficult and will always involve some extra thought and effort. However it can become a much more comfortable process for all concerned if attention is paid to constructing a better communication environment.

COMMUNICATIVE ENVIRONMENTS

An environmental approach to the rehabilitation of communication disordered people requires us to create a stimulating environment where there is something worth talking about as well as the opportunity to talk. In such an environment the communication disordered person carries some responsibility for communicating. There is less need for other people to speak on his behalf all the time because their communication skills have adapted to the environment to make his own performance as effective as possible.

It is notoriously difficult for clients to generalize skills which have been acquired in the safety of a rehabilitation clinic to a wider environment. For instance, the speech of someone who has slurred speech (dysarthria) will greatly improve when he is speaking one to one with a therapist who helps him monitor his speech and reminds him to use strategies that improve his intelligibility (such as slowing the rate of speech and splitting up long words into syllables). This same client will then walk out of the room and automatically greet friends in the corridor with speech which is dramatically reduced in intelligibility. I term this phenomenon *the corridor effect* and it is observed to a greater or lesser extent in most communication disorders.

Poor generalization is a problem that the client often never successfully overcomes and so we have a situation where he is capable of improving his performance considerably in certain special situations but does not do this in everyday interactions. His functional performance remains permanently below the level he might otherwise expect to achieve given his residual formal abilities. Is such a client simply being lazy and uncooperative, bearing in mind that most people in this situation are desperate to improve their ability, or is there something else that accounts for this inconsistency or corridor effect? Perhaps the likely explanation requires us to consider not just what the client is or is not doing, but what the therapist is contributing to the exchange. The client's superior performance in the clinic setting occurs solely because the therapist is able to create a micro-environment which is tailor-made to be the very best for that client's communicative needs. Such an assumption makes sense because any skills which the client has acquired at this stage are bound to be fragile and only able to survive in a sympathetic milieu where he has everything going for him. Clients will repeatedly assert how much easier and enjoyable they find it to talk to a therapist than with other people. This is not because therapists are better interpreters but because there is more equal participation. The therapist knows how to modify the physical, emotional and linguistic environments from minute to minute in order to help. By linguistic environment I mean the therapist modifies his/her own speech output, for example by slowing the rate of speech, using simpler sentence structures, or sticking to 'here and now' concepts rather than abstract ones.

Communication therapists themselves are well aware of the corridor effect but even they tend not to take full advantage of the implications. They often see it as representing their own lack of expertise in enabling the patient to take his abilities outside the clinic, rather than as an indication of how their own specialized communication skills are instrumental in inducing the temporary improvement.

The skills necessary to do this can be learned by anyone and theoretically the whole of the client's environment can be modified to maximize his performance. The aim of doing so is not to cure or rehabilitate the patient, as cure is usually not possible and rehabilitation needs the direction of the relevant professionals, but rather to make sure the client has the best possible chance of communicating well. Where an environmental approach is used this becomes the permanent responsibility of everyone with whom the client subsequently comes into contact and extends well beyond any active period of rehabilitation.

THE COMMUNICATION CYCLE

When we speak to someone with a communication handicap we usually feel uncomfortable as a result of the feelings that get in the way of all the useful things we might otherwise attempt to do.

A role-play exercise I have often used in workshops gives participants the experience of not being able to communicate adequately by allocating severe restrictions to their speech. The group then shares and examines the feelings generated by the experience. Here is a typical set of responses to the exercise:

AS A SPEAKER I FELT:	AS A LISTENER I FELT:
– frustrated	– it was hard work
– embarrassed	– annoyed
– irritated	– frustrated
– he could have helped me more	– exasperated
	– tired
– I wanted to explain my 'rules'	– embarrassed
	– annoyed with myself
– tired	– inadequate
– it was hard work	– it would have helped to know his problem
– I wanted to give up	
– annoyed with self	– it was time-consuming
– inadequate	– impatient
– it was hard to concentrate	– it was hard to concentrate

It is obvious that the two lists are similar if not identical, indicating

36

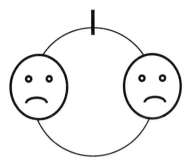

Fig. 2.2 The communication cycle. When it is broken at any point neither participant can experience easy communication.

(perhaps surprisingly) that both speakers and listeners are simultaneously struggling with the same feelings. In the case of the normal speaker all these rather negative feelings get in the way of any useful adaptive behaviour.

The presence of such feelings is probably a consequence of the two-way nature of communication (Fig. 2.2). For successful communication to occur all parts of the communication cycle need to be working normally. If our conversational partner is unable to communicate well, our own ability to communicate will be adversely affected and no matter how competent a communicator we are, we will still not be able to have a normal interaction. In other words **we** are directly experiencing a communication handicap. This is somewhat different from confronting other handicaps. When pushing someone in a wheelchair, there may be places you cannot take that person but your own ability to walk is unaffected. Thus the negative feelings around when talking to someone with a communication handicap are the result of both parties simultaneously struggling with a deficit in their performance.

As we have already suggested, strategies that facilitate communication can be employed to make the exchange easier and to build up the confidence of both parties. Some of these are common to all communication handicaps and are described below. Where strategies are specific to a particular disorder, they are considered in later chapters alongside that disorder.

**IMPROVING COMMUNICATION WITH SOMEONE WHO HAS A
COMMUNICATION DISORDER**

1. Always include the person in conversations. If nothing else this can be done with eye contact and facial expression. If you know they cannot answer a question, address the query directly and then look to a third party for the answer.
2. Choose somewhere quiet and peaceful to talk wherever possible. This gives both of you an opportunity to concentrate and not be distracted.
3. Do one thing at a time. This saves the person having to compete for your attention. Make it obvious that you are focusing on the conversation, perhaps by sitting down or at least standing still. Many communication disordered people cannot walk and talk at the same time.
4. Don't shout. This is counterproductive in nearly all instances unless there is a mild hearing loss. It distorts normal patterns of lip movement, thus removing a useful source of clues.
5. Give time. Disguise any feelings you may have of being in a hurry. Impatience on your part will have a negative effect on the other's speech.
6. Look at the person you're talking to. This will show you are attending, give you clues about his messages and enable you to lip read. We all lip read each other in the normal course of events, it is not a strategy that is only used by deaf people.
7. Don't criticize. He is likely to be his own most severe critic.
8. Don't pretend to understand. He will eventually realize that you don't and draw the inevitable conclusion that you are not interested. In any case, if you do not tell him that you are not understanding he cannot make any effort to help you.
9. Offer suggestions as to what you think has been said. This must be done with tact and care if despite repetitions you are still not clear. Make sure you give him an opportunity to indicate whether you have guessed correctly or not.
10. Remember to smile. When concentrating on all the above points it is easy to end up looking severe and unfriendly. Make sure you are giving the messages you wish to.

When normal speakers are first introduced to the idea of modifying their communication they sometimes fear it can only be done at the expense of natural sincerity and spontaneity. Such an anxiety is normal and understandable but not necessarily valid. We always feel self-conscious and awkward when trying out any new skill or way of behaving. Initially we have to split the behaviour into its component parts and practise them as separate activities. Only as we become more *au fait* with the discrete manoeuvres can we begin to integrate them. Eventually they become automatic and easy. As I drive my car I am not conscious of changing gear, steering or moving my right foot from the accelerator to the brake, although when I was learning to drive all these things seemed very cumbersome and difficult. Not any more. However, I recently had to drive a minibus with 12 people in it and once again became acutely aware of all the component activities involved in driving because the context had changed and I was having to accommodate those changes. I was also convinced that all the passengers must be equally aware of my lack of familiarity with the vehicle. If I drove a minibus regularly it would soon become as easy as driving my car, and enjoyable as well. So it is when adapting a language style. Initially awkward in each new context, with practice, not to mention some success, we can reach a stage where it once again feels natural, honest and spontaneous.

RIGHT OR LUXURY?

Without doubt, taking time to employ successful communication strategies can dramatically improve the quality of conversations for communication disordered clients, but even so any exchange will still take longer than it would with a normal person. Aspects of physical care such as giving appointments, instructions about health care and getting accurate information for diagnostic purposes all have to be attended to eventually, and in fact not to do so results in wasted time and money and may even be downright dangerous. Adequate attention must also be given to psychological care to prevent the inevitable isolation and likelihood of depression. It is vital for the client to be socially included. Unfortunately, because this takes time and because communication disordered people are easy clients to avoid, this frequently does not happen.

Nurses who genuinely want to help often say that they would like to spend more time with their communication disordered patients but that the realities of a busy ward make this impractical. All health professionals are busy people and I used to respond to this challenge by pointing out that such clients are going to be time-consuming anyway and that if communication does not occur satisfactorily in the short term it will take up even more time in the long term. Consequently it makes sense to do it well the first time round and save the necessity for repeated attempts. I now regard the issue in a rather different light. Surely the client is entitled to the extra time as a right rather than as a luxury or as an optional extra which is metered out if the circumstances are favourable. If taking the time to employ successful communication strategies alleviates the client's difficulties, then it is his right to have it. The problem of how to provide the time is one for the professionals to sort out. A comparison can be made with the allocation of surgical and drug treatments, where it is accepted that within reason the client receives the appropriate treatment. The professionals are responsible for organizing and providing this even though resources may be limited.

3

The normal development of language, articulation and phonology

LANGUAGE

We use language to structure our thoughts and to convey those thoughts to others. Language is extremely complex and our use of it is normally extensive and automatic. How we learn and develop the ability to use such an intricate system of symbols has long fascinated linguists, communication therapists, psychologists and others. Theories of language acquisition abound but whatever the abstract differences between them, the stages apparent in the developing child's use of language can be described.

Vocabulary

Vocabulary is acquired quickly. At 12 months the average child will understand a few words related to his immediate environment such as the names of family members and parts of the body. A little later he will begin to produce those same words. At this early stage, the concepts the child links to the labels do not exactly match those of an adult. This is demonstrated by the 12-month old child who refers to all men as 'daddy'. It is not a fault in the child's language, he is merely matching the label to what he knows of the world, namely that a big male person is called 'daddy'. He then over-extends the use of that label to other similar people. By 5 years of age the child understands and is capable of using several thousand verbal labels. In addition he will realize that certain items possess similar characteristics and that words exist which recognize this, so 'pig,' 'horse','cow' and 'lion' are all 'animals'. This growing awareness is coupled with a developing ability to use several words in order to describe a specific idea or object, e.g. a 'bed' is 'soft' and used for 'sleeping'.

Comprehension

At 1 year of age the child responds primarily to simple phrases, particularly those which are used routinely and in familiar situations, e.g. 'Wave bye bye' as the child is leaving a room. He is also just beginning to pick out a familiar word when it is heard in a longer sentence. He is able to interpret this single word and to respond fairly accurately, e.g. 'We're going to the shops now so put your coat on'. At this stage the child does not understand every word in the sentence, but combines his knowledge of the word such as it is, with his understanding of the context in order to respond. He knows what a coat is and that there are a limited number of things you can do with coats.

By the age of 5 years the child has acquired knowledge of a vast amount of oral language so that:

1. Verbal labels for concepts of size, colour, shape and position are understood.
2. Question forms such as why, when, where and who are known.
3. Tense markers and their effect on the meaning of a sentence are recognized. The child realizes that someone saying 'We had an ice-cream yesterday' means something quite different from 'We'll have an ice-cream now'.
4. There is an ability to understand and use increasingly complex language structures, e.g. 'Yesterday I ate some biscuits because I was very hungry'.
5. The child is able to integrate the complex skills involved in concentrating, listening and understanding a story and will later be able to answer questions on it and later still even formulate a version of his own.

Expression

The development of expressive language roughly parallels that of receptive or comprehension skills. In general a child will always understand more than he is able to use. Around the first birthday a few single words will begin to appear but as has already been described, the use of the label will be broad so that 'duck' may be applied to any bird. This over-extension of labels gradually reduces as the child's vocabulary grows.

By the time he is 5 years old the child can compile and use complicated sentences:

'If I sit on my chair while I eat my tea can I watch television later?'

Purpose

In addition to the actual development of comprehension and use of language forms, the child must also learn how language changes depending on the context and desired outcome. This involves the following.

The development of turn-taking skills

Taking turns is a vital feature in the organization of a conversation. A young child is poor at taking turns and will speak across another person. Initially he will be told 'Don't speak when I'm speaking' but he will gradually learn to recognize the more subtle cues which indicate when it is acceptable for him to respond. He will also become aware of his obligation to take up his turn in a conversation.

Relevance

In a conversation involving two adults, each speaker will have responsibility for making sure that what he says is relevant to what has gone before. This is something a young child has to learn to do. An 18-month old child may say whatever he feels like, whether it is relevant or not, but by 5 years of age he will try hard to be relevant.

Use of language

The child learns that language can be used in different forms, among others, to request, socialize, deny and question. He also learns to use language indirectly, e.g.

'Do you know mummy, I haven't had an ice-cream all week.'

Language styles

Different language styles such as humour and polite speech are appropriate at different times depending on the situation. At 24 months a child will demand 'Want drink', whereas at 5 years old he will say 'Can I have a drink please?'

In spoken language sounds convey meaning. If the correct sounds are not used, or are used in the wrong order then the speaker will find it hard to make himself understood. Before we can appreciate the problems someone may have with the mechanics of speaking, it is necessary to understand the difference between being able to make a single sound and being able to use that sound in conjunction with other sounds. The former process is termed articulation and the latter phonology.

ARTICULATION

At about 6 months a baby begins to practise the oral movements he will eventually need for sound production. This sound play or babbling involves making single sounds such as 'da', and strings of sounds 'dadadada'. It is important to realize that, at this stage, the child is only practising the mechanics of sound production and is not using the sounds to convey meaning.

Many muscles are used in the process of making sounds and in some cases the difference between one sound and another is slight and achieved by subtle but complex oral movements. Lips, teeth, tongue, hard and soft palate, pharynx and the vocal cords are all employed to generate sounds and to differentiate one from another. The baby has to learn accurately to reproduce all the sounds that are ultimately going to be used in his own language. No one language uses all the noises it is possible to make with the human articulatory system. Neither the French nor Asian 'r' sounds appear in spoken English and some African languages use clicking sounds that do not exist in English.

When individual sounds are linked together as in words, the oral movements become even more complex and a child learns the combinations of manoeuvres which will enable him accurately to move from one sound to another. As he gets older he will be able to master more and more complicated movements and hence will eventually be able to make sounds such as 'ch, x, sk, gl, skr'.

Because we are used to reading we tend to think of sounds as discrete items in the same way as letters, but in speech sounds in the same or adjacent words influence and change each other. How the sound is actually produced will depend on whereabouts it appears in the word and what sounds occur on either side of it. This effect can sometimes interfere with the production of newly acquired sounds in the young child.

Consider the consonants /k/ and /t/. (The symbols used for the sound are the phonetic representations of the sounds to avoid confusion with the alphabet letter names 'kay' and 'tee'.) /k/ is formed by touching the soft palate with the back of the tongue (try it and see), whereas /t/ is formed by touching the hard palate with the front of the tongue (Fig. 3.1). If a child is attempting to say a word beginning with /k/ he is more likely to be successful if the preceding sound is also made somewhere at the back of the mouth. The vowel 'a' as in 'car' falls into this category whereas the vowel 'ee' is made at the front of the mouth. Hence it is easier for the child to say 'car' than 'key' despite the fact that the words begin with the same sound. In fact a young child trying to say 'key' will often come out with 'tee' because the front vowel 'ee' brings the consonant forward as well. As the normal child matures this distortion disappears.

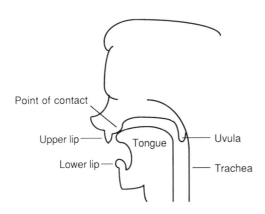

Fig. 3.1 The position of the articulators for the production of /t/.

PHONOLOGY

If one digit in a telephone number is changed, the whole number is then different. And there will be varying consequences if that wrong number is used with the original intention. So our spoken language is dependent upon our ability to produce and interpret patterns of sound. It is the pattern that gives us the meaning, not the individual items. Each particular component has to be correct or the meaning of the word and perhaps the whole sentence or whole communication is changed. As children each of us has to learn the patterns of sound that occur in our own language.

Certain characteristics of sounds serve as special markers which enable us to hear the difference between one sound and another and establish what the patterns are. These markers are known as sound contrasts. If a person has poor awareness of these characteristics it will also be difficult for them to produce the contrasts themselves. Some of these marker features are described below, (The sound system of any language includes both vowels and consonants but in this description we will consider only the consonants.)

Place of articulation

The articulators used to make the sound will determine where in the mouth that sound is made.

e.g.	/p/	–	lips (front)
	/th/	–	tongue + teeth (front)
	/t/	–	tongue + hard palate (front)
	/k/	–	tongue + soft palate (back)
	/f/	–	lips and teeth (front)

Some people can produce accurate sounds when they occur singly but are not able to combine sounds in the right patterns needed for correct words and sentences. This is a normal feature of phonological development. If it persists beyond certain development points then that child is said to have a phonological disorder. A young child may be able to say the sound /k/ correctly when asked, but when talking use the sound /t/ instead.

46

Thus: 'car' becomes 'tar'
'cat' becomes 'tat'
'cow' becomes 'tow'

This happens because the child has not yet managed to identify what makes the difference between /k/ and /t/. As already described, /k/ is made by using the back of the tongue to touch the soft palate and temporarily stop the flow of air out through the mouth, rather than placing the tip of the tongue against the hard palate as we do for /t/. Hence /k/ is made at the back of the mouth and /t/ nearer the front. In other words the place in the mouth at which the sound is made is different for these two sounds.

Manner of articulation

Nasality

Here the airstream is prevented from escaping through the mouth by closing the oral cavity as for the sound /m/. The closure occurs at the lips and at the same time the soft palate is lowered to enable the airstream to pass through and into the nasal cavity (Fig. 3.2). Thus we are able to contrast oral and nasal sounds. Most sounds need an oral airstream. The nasals used in English are /m/ and /n/ and the 'ng' sound as heard at the end of 'going' (unless the speaker has an accent where the /g/ is pronounced, as for example in the Manchester and Birmingham areas of England).

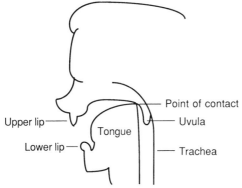

Fig. 3.2 The position of the articulators for the production of /k/.

Plosion

The airstream is allowed to pass through the mouth but is temporarily blocked by the articulators. Air pressure builds up behind the block until the articulators are suddenly moved apart, releasing a burst of air. So for /p/ the lips are held together against the air which is being pushed through the mouth, and then suddenly released. Plosives include /p,b,t,d,k,g/. Trying holding your hand in front of your mouth and saying these sounds. Each time you will feel a puff of air released on your hand.

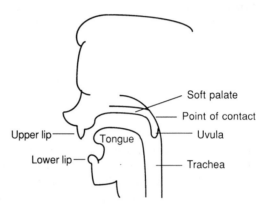

Fig. 3.3 Position of the uvula for oral sounds.

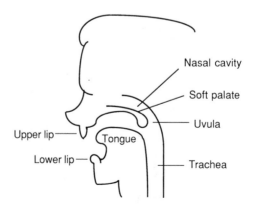

Fig. 3.4 The position of the uvula for nasal sounds.

Friction

Here the articulators are almost closed but not quite and thus only a narrow column of air is allowed to pass through the mouth. This causes turbulence in the airstream which we auditorily perceive as friction. Fricatives include s,z,sh,f,v,th.

Voice

Some sounds require the vocal cords to be vibrating, others do not. This means some sounds are voiced and others voiceless. Sometimes the only difference between one sound and another is the amount of voicing present.

The sound /s/ is made by forcing an oral airstream through a narrow channel between the front of the tongue and the hard palate and so is /z/. However /z/ is accompanied by vocal cord vibration and /s/ is not. Place your fingers lightly over your larynx and say 'sss' and then 'zzz'. You will feel a vibration in your throat with the latter indicating that your vocal cords are being used. The pairs of sounds below are made in an identical way except for the voicing:

voiceless	:	voiced
p	:	b
t	:	d
k	:	g
f	:	v
s	:	z
ch	:	j

We have to learn how to employ all the above markers in order to convey meaning. For example the words 'pea' and 'bee' are contrasted solely by the fact that the first sound in 'bee' is voiced. Without that contrast, only one of the two words can be produced and without further information the listener cannot tell which of the two is the intended word.

IMPROVING YOUR COMMUNICATION WITH CHILDREN

We can modify the way we talk to children to enhance the interaction just as we can with adults. The following pointers are useful when talking to any child, whether they have a communication problem or not.

1. Check out your spacing.
With children this mainly involves the vertical spacing. Ideally you need to have your eyes at the same level as the child's. This may mean you have to crouch down but it becomes less intimidating for him.

2. Be careful with questions.
Don't ask too many or place the child in a situation where there is a lot of pressure for him to answer 'correctly' in front of other people.

3. Try to gauge the level of language that he is likely to understand and simplify sentences where possible. With young children try and keep topics to the here and now rather than using very abstract concepts.

4. Be aware of turn-taking.
Allow pauses for the child to respond and wait for him to finish what he's saying before you go on to something else. Being interrupted may make it hard for him to keep the thread of what he is saying.

5. Concentrate on one thing at a time.
If he is engrossed in something else or if there are a number of distractions, very young children will find it difficult to absorb what you say. Doing two things at once in this way becomes easier as the child grows older.

6. Avoid 'demand speech'.
Adults often demand speech of children as a way of encouraging them to talk and join in conversations. The child is told when to speak and what to say: 'Say hello.' 'Say you're sorry.' 'Tell daddy what you did this morning.' 'Tell Doreen where we're going now.' This puts a great pressure on the child to perform. It is better to encourage conversation in response to a comment. 'We went to see Grandma today . . .' leaves the child a choice as to whether he responds or not.

7. Give time.
Children may need longer to formulate what they want to say, as well as to make sense of what you have just said. Pace the conversation more slowly than you would with an adult.

8.   Do not force repetitions.
It is normal for the child to make some errors in his pronunciation.
If you wish to correct him, you need only give him a correct
model without making him practise it.

child: 'Daniel go in tar.'
adult: 'In the car. Yes, we're going when I've found my purse.'

9.   Give feedback.
Children need feedback in a conversation just as much as adults.
Eye-contact, smiles and nods all encourage him and give him
confidence.

THE EFFECT OF AGEING ON COMMUNICATION

As a person gets older we can observe changes in comprehension,
expression and the way language is used, as well as changes in
speech and voice quality (Gravell, 1988). Chronological age is
not always a reliable indicator of someone's mental and physical
performance; physiologically some people age faster than others.
Perceptual and sensory changes have a significant effect on
communication and can be either peripheral or central. There
seems to be a decreasing sensitivity in vision, hearing, taste and
smell with increasing age. Hearing impairment is a particularly
common cause of reduced communicative ability among the
elderly. Ageing also makes it harder for us to acquire and store
new information in our memory, either as a result of a reduced
ability to encode material or to retrieve it. Attention skills are
often reported as being reduced in older people but this is not
proven. Learning is influenced by many things but in general older
people find it harder to learn new things. Thus we can expect to
see a decline in comprehension and expressive language ability.
Changes in the respiratory system make it harder to control the
breath supply for speech and hence there are changes in voice
quality and pitch. Male voices have a tendency towards a higher
pitch with increasing age and so there is a less marked difference
between male and female pitch ranges. There is a higher incidence
of diseases such as Parkinson's disease and CVAs among the
elderly which carry specific communication deficits (Broe *et al.*,
1976).
Some tests of language and communicative ability allow for this

normal effect of ageing and have some means of adjusting the raw scores to give a more realistic interpretation of the data gained. This prevents people being diagnosed as dysphasic just because they have reached a certain age.

A diagnosis of a specific communication problem in an elderly person would of course take the normal changes due to age into account.

4

Problems in speech and language development

The complex language skills already outlined are normally well established by the age of five. When things do not go smoothly the nature of the consequent difficulties can be divided into two main groups, language delay and language disorder.

LANGUAGE DELAY

Here the skills emerge in the normal developmental order but at a slower rate. The delay may be in all areas of language or in any one or more of these areas. A delay in language development may be associated with a more general developmental delay or it may be an isolated feature of the child's maturation. In some cases the aetiology of the delay may be linked with some other problem such as a hearing loss, adverse environmental conditions or emotional trauma.

LANGUAGE DISORDER

One or more of the component skills may fail to appear or may appear very slowly. There may be deviations from, and distortions of, a normal pattern. When a diagnosis of language disorder is made the problem is frequently a specific one with no associated general developmental delay. A severe disorder in language may have significant implications for subsequent school progress and social integration.

Types of language disorder include the following.

Word-finding problems

A child may have a good understanding of verbal labels but have extreme difficulty in recalling those labels for his own use. He may circumlocate the word he intends:

e.g. CHAIR '. . . um, you sit on it, it's got legs.'

or offer a word with a similar meaning

e.g. CHAIR becomes STOOL

or a word with similar sounds

e.g. CHAIR becomes CHIMNEY

These strategies can seriously disrupt the flow of the child's language and will undoubtedly affect the way in which he is perceived by those around him.

Comprehension problems

The child may find it difficult to interpret language that he hears. The problem may be mild – perhaps he is not able to understand the use of tenses – or so severe as to render meaningless any language he hears.

Expression

The child may not be able to perceive the patterns necessary for forming meaningful language. Again the problem may be either mild or severe enough to restrict him to single words. It may even prevent him from speaking at all.

Semantic-pragmatic language functions

The child may find it hard to use language appropriately in context. He may be unable to make his language relevant to what has gone before. He may interpret language literally and therefore may not understand humour, so that when told 'It's raining cats and dogs,' he may expect to see animals falling from the sky.

THE EFFECTS OF LANGUAGE DELAY AND DISORDER

Although a language delay or disorder is often not accompanied by other types of handicap its effect on the child and those around him may be far more wide reaching than is usually appreciated.

Effects which involve the family

Guilt

Parents of a language handicapped child often experience guilt, believing they are somehow responsible for the child's problem and for not being able to resolve it.

Rejection of the problem

Some parents find it hard to accept that their child actually has a difficulty. Positive help in enabling them to adjust is essential both in order to establish a basis for therapy and to provide a secure, accepting and understanding family environment for the child.

Rejection of the child

This is a less common reaction but nevertheless it does occur. The establishment and maintenance of all relationships are heavily dependent on communication and the relationship between a parent and a child who has a communication disorder can suffer. Counselling helps to minimize potential damage both for the parents and the child.

Siblings

Siblings of the affected child may receive less attention from the parents or have unrealistic expectations placed on them, or be scapegoated by the family. They may avoid interaction with the language handicapped child and older siblings may overindulge him/her (Rollin, 1987).

Effects which involve the peer group

A child with impaired language skills will find it difficult to relate to siblings and peers. His responses to language, or his own use of language, may differ from those of his peers and mark him as different. The child can easily become shy, withdrawn, isolated and prone to temper tantrums. These behaviours only serve to mark the child still further.

It is important to create an accepting environment around the child. At the same time he needs to be presented with challenges and actively integrated with his peers.

IMPLICATIONS FOR EDUCATION

It is easy to assume that a child with communication difficulties has accompanying cognitive problems but this is not necessarily true. Teachers need to be advised as to the specific nature of the language handicap so that appropriate management of the child can be maintained at school. The general implications for the child's schooling will depend upon the type of disability he presents. Skills which involve language such as reading may well be affected. In severe cases a child may need special schooling related to his specific language disability and placement in a language unit or school for children with communication problems may be advisable. In Britain there are now a number of residential schools nationwide and most large centres have one or more language units attached to ordinary schools. A short placement in such a school or unit is often followed by a return to mainstream education. However it is usual and desirable that children with mild or moderate language problems be maintained in mainstream schools.

REMEDIATION OF LANGUAGE DELAY AND DISORDER

A child who is diagnosed as having a language disability will need communication therapy. Management will then be affected by the age of the child, severity of the disorder and by the insight and motivation of the family. Any direct therapy with the child should always involve family counselling and sometimes active teaching of the parents to enable them to participate in therapy programmes.

Management options might include:

Intensive therapy: several hours a day for blocks of 2–3 weeks.
Regular therapy: attendance once a week lasting from a few weeks to several years.
Periodic review: say every 3–6 months. This may be used in conjunction with language programmes carried out by the family at home.

Some disorders respond better than others to intervention. A language handicap is obviously compounded by any associated learning disability. Where the problem is that of a language delay and there is no accompanying general developmental delay, normal language can be expected to develop eventually. If there is a general developmental delay then it is unlikely that normal language levels will ever be reached.

For the child with a language disorder the prognosis is much more variable and the more severe the presenting symptoms, the less the likelihood of the problems resolving completely. Severe language difficulties may persist throughout adult life but children with milder ones may achieve normal language at some point. For children in the former category specialized schooling may be necessary to maximize their potential

COMMON PROBLEMS IN ARTICULATION

If a child has an articulation problem there will usually be an identifiable aetiology such as cleft palate, hearing loss or a neurological deficit, but they may not always have an identifiable pathology. Sounds and combinations of sounds appear in a more or less predictable sequence and a child can be expected to have acquired particular sounds by certain stages in his development. Thus any slowness or deviation from the expected can be detected. It is almost impossible to discuss articulation deficits (those involving the production of isolated sounds), without also considering the effect on phonology and how sounds are used in conjunction with other sounds.

Lisps

It is probably worth considering this particular articulation problem here because of its common presentation in children. Fricatives are often problematic because in articulatory terms they are complex sounds and some of the last to appear developmentally. The term fricative refers to the fact that the sound is produced by friction as air is forced between the articulators. So /s/ is made by pushing an airstream through a narrow groove formed by the front of the tongue and the hard palate. Other fricatives include /f/ and /th/. The commonly presenting /s/ problems are when the sound is made too far forward in the mouth (dentalized), too far back (palatalized) or when air is allowed to escape round the sides of the tongue (producing a lateral /s/). It is hard to pinpoint reasons for the development of a lisp and there is no clear pattern to link factors such as dentition or jaw structure.

A dental /s/ often disappears on its own by the age of seven years old and beyond this age stands a good chance of resolution even in adulthood. Adults have often adjusted to their lisp and are not bothered by it sufficiently to seek therapy but occasionally candidates for careers such as the police force or those that carry a high level of speaking performance are asked to remedy their articulation. A lateral /s/ is much more intransigent and rarely goes without remediation and hence intervention begins earlier.

PHONOLOGICAL DISORDERS

We have seen how, in order to convey meaning, the child must learn which set of sounds are used and which features mark the differences between one sound and another in his language. The words 'town' and 'down' are contrasted solely by the fact that the first sound in 'down' is voiced. If a child is not able to use that contrast he will only be able to produce one of the two words and without further information it is not possible for the listener to know which of the two words the child is wanting to say.

The fewer the contrasts used, the more restricted the set of sounds available to the child. As sounds convey meaning, the child who has a very restricted sound system will have considerable difficulty in making himself understood.

The aetiology of phonological disorders is not always as clear as that of articulation disorders and to complicate things further the relation between articulation and phonology is more complex than is at first apparent. Often with a phonological problem the pattern is one of no obvious physiological/anatomical deficit and usually there is:

• normal hearing;
• no anatomical or physiological abnormality of oral structures;
• no major neurological deficit relating to speech production;
• intellectual development within a range adequate for normal acquisition of speech and language, i.e. may include some children with learning difficulties;
• comprehension is appropriate for the age of the child;
• no evidence of inadequate interpersonal language experience.

As with language disorder, phonological disorders fall into two main categories. In delayed phonology the development of a sound system follows a normal pattern but occurs at a slower than normal rate. In deviant phonology the pattern of development is unusual and/or idiosyncratic. Common speech characteristics of children who have phonological disorders are:

• a restricted range of consonants, both in number and variety;
• few indications of differences between sounds, with some of the features that are normally used to make sound contrasts not being employed at all. Some non-English sounds present in speech;
• few combinations or clusters of consonants are used, e.g. sm/ st/fl/pl/kr/;
• sounds at the end of words are often omitted so CAP becomes 'CA-'; BUS becomes 'BU-'.

REMEDIATION OF PHONOLOGICAL DISORDERS

Early referral to a communication therapist is necessary and a detailed assessment is needed to determine a specific description of the child's problem. Listening to a large sample of conversation gives much more information than asking the child to perform single words. The child must then become aware of how his sound system should operate as well as how individual sounds are made.

Treatment may take place over a period of months and the child will be seen either on his own or in a group. Parental involvement is essential and the higher their commitment to the treatment programme, the more likely the problems are to resolve. Parents may be expected to work daily with their child. Factors such as time of referral, transient hearing loss and intelligence will affect the rate of progress.

Children with only mild degrees of phonological delay may respond to working on programmes at home and require only occasional visits to a communication therapist. Those with severe difficulties who may be virtually unintelligible to anyone outside their immediate family may need to attend clinics regularly, maybe once a week initially and then less frequently for up to five years. If a child does not receive help he may be so frustrated by repeatedly unsuccessful attempts to communicate that he gives up or becomes disruptive. It is important that symptoms of distress such as withdrawal, temper tantrums and nocturnal enuresis are prevented or alleviated.

Inadequate phonology can affect social as well as language developments for it deters the child from experimenting with people and relationships. Although some children who are not treated may eventually acquire normal speech spontaneously, this inevitably occurs at the expense of early social, emotional and intellectual development.

MARKERS OF SPEECH AND LANGUAGE DEVELOPMENT

The presence or absence of particular features in the child's speech at a given age suggests cause for concern.

Expression

By 12 months – he doesn't produce any consonants (m, n, p, b, t, d, k, g) or raspberries.
– doesn't produce any longer vowel type sounds.
– doesn't put words and consonants together: 'ma', 'ba', 'mamamama'.
12–18 months – doesn't use nonsense speech (jargon).
By 18 months – does use jargon but no sign of words emerging.
By 24 months – there are no recognizable words.

By 32 months	–	does not combine two words: 'Make juice.' 'Mummy gone.'
By 3 years	–	there are no sentences of three or more words.
	–	the first consonant in words is omitted: shoe becomes '. . . oo' fish becomes '. . . ish' me becomes '. . . ee'
	–	speech is hard to understand. By three years 75% of a child's speech should be intelligible.
By 4 years	–	consonants are missed off the end of words: seat becomes 'sea..' dog becomes 'do . . .' cat becomes 'ca . . .'
After 4 years	–	there are poorly formed sentences which are confusing or telegraphic in style.
	–	there are word reversals: going home becomes 'home going'.
5 years	–	there are immature combinations of sounds used in place of complex ones.
At any age	–	the child experiences embarrassment or disturbed feelings about speech.

Comprehension

6–12 months	–	the child fails to respond to the voices of family members especially after periods of absence when that member is still out of sight and not touching the infant.
	–	the child fails to respond to environmental sounds in the absence of a hearing loss.
By 18 months	–	the child does not understand common words and simple commands.
12–24 months	–	there is a failure to indicate a few familiar objects or people when those objects are named or marked by gesture.
24–30 months	–	familiar objects and people are not pointed to when they are named without the cue of gestures.
24–36 months	–	people comment that the child is slow and

takes a long time to catch on to what has been said.

CLEFT PALATE

Each year 1500 children are born in Great Britain with congenital clefts of the lip and palate. This is about one in 600 births. Clefts can be classified as:

1. Cleft lip only, with or without involvement of the alveolus;
2. Unilateral cleft lip and palate involving both hard and soft palates;
3. Bilateral cleft lip and palate involving both hard and soft palates;
4. Cleft palate involving soft palate only or both hard and soft palates.

Children born with an isolated cleft lip do not normally develop speech or language deficits whereas those born with cleft palate (with or without a cleft lip) are at risk of developing communication problems.

Language

The child may be slow to use language (delay) or he may develop abnormal patterns of language use (disorder). Evidence suggests cleft palate children use shorter and less complex sentences than normal children of the same age. This may be due to:

Hearing impairment

An accompanying catarrhal hearing loss is very common.

Reduced use of language

A child with unintelligible speech may well cut down on the actual amount of speaking he does in order to make it easier to be understood.

Parental reactions

Parents will be upset by the birth of a handicapped child and may be overprotective. If they continually anticipate the child's needs and he never has to ask for anything he wants, then language development will be slow. In addition the parents may expect their child to be a poor communicator and therefore accept immature language from him.

Hospitalization

Usually primary and some secondary surgery takes place during the first five years. As this period is also critical for language and social development, traumatic events occurring during this time can have detrimental effects on the child's ability to learn and use language.

Phonology and articulation

The physical abnormalities of the palate may make it impossible for the child to produce certain sounds accurately. If he is unable to make these sounds easily he will start to substitute other easier sounds in their place or omit sounds altogether. These two effects will make his speech difficult if not impossible to understand. Such articulation and phonological errors may be caused or exacerbated by:

a. Hearing impairment.

b. Dentition/occlusion.
Badly placed teeth can restrict and distort tongue movements. In Pierre-Robin syndrome there may be disproportion of the maxillary and mandibular arches and a resultant difficulty in closing the lips.

c. Palatal incompetence.
Here, despite surgery, the palate cannot move sufficiently to make contact with the back wall of the pharynx and is unable completely to block off the nasal passages. As a consequence air escapes into the nasal cavity and pharynx, the oral/nasal contrast cannot be made accurately and air can often be heard escaping down the nose (nasal escape). The greater the palatal incompetence the worse the articulation will be.

d.   Poor sucking and feeding patterns.

Abnormal tongue movements are likely to be adopted by the infant who has an unrepaired cleft, in an effort to compensate when feeding. This gives a poor basis for speech.

The combined result of the above means that some typical articulation and phonological errors are associated with cleft palate. Sounds normally made at the front of the mouth are replaced by sounds normally made at the back.

> e.g.   /t/ is produced as /k/ therefore TAP becomes 'KAP'
>   /d/ is produced as /g/ therefore DOG becomes 'GOG'

In the first example the incorrect though real word 'CAP' is accidentally produced, whereas in the second case a nonsense word 'GOG' is formed.

Oral sounds involving air being passed through the mouth are replaced by nasals as the child's palate is not able to separate the oral and nasal cavities.

> e.g.   /b/ is produced as /m/ therefore BALL becomes 'MALL'
>   /d/ is produced as /n/ therefore DAY becomes 'NAY'

Sounds which are produced with the tip of the tongue are difficult for the child with a cleft palate to make. Such sounds would include /t/d/s/z/sh/. In addition consonants are often missed off the ends of words in cleft palate speech.

> BED becomes 'BE-'
> SHIP becomes 'SHI-'

The combined effects of the above errors severely limit the child's intelligibility.

Voice

The actual sound of the voice may be different from that of a normal child. Generally the speech is characterized by hypernasality (too much nasal resonance), but less commonly there can be hyponasality (too little resonance). Nasal escape is often associated with hypernasality when the audible emission of air can be heard on consonant sounds. There may also be some vocal hoarseness due to compensatory attempts to overcome the hypernasality.

Feeding

Almost all babies with anything other than a very minor cleft have some difficulty feeding, particularly if the cleft is complete and involves the lip as well as the hard and soft palates. The baby is not able to generate the negative pressure within the mouth which is necessary for sucking and stimulating a flow of milk from either a breast or bottle. The back of the tongue may hump in an attempt to achieve this. Feeding takes a long time and the baby can become exhausted before the meal is finished.

Management of cleft palate

This is carried out by a team which may comprise a plastic surgeon, paediatrician, orthodontist, communication therapist, ENT consultant, parents, audiologist and nursing staff. Involvement of some team members may continue well into teenage years. The child will need regular help with communication for up to five years and less regularly as he grows older.

Good feeding habits must be established from birth as this may affect the child's ability to produce speech sounds later on. Sucking should be encouraged whenever possible and some bottle teats are more useful than others.

Most centres where cleft palate surgery is carried out hold regular clinics where the child is reviewed regularly by all the specialists and joint recommendations are made. Hearing tests will also need to be carried out at regular intervals. Initially speech and language intervention is aimed at the prevention of bad habits. Advice is given to encourage babbling and pre-verbal skills. Regular help will help correct faulty articulation and stimulate language production.

In the older cleft palate child the most obvious remaining problem is usually excessive hypernasality and further surgery may be necessary to correct this. The procedure involves stitching a flap of tissue taken from the posterior pharyngeal wall onto the soft palate (posterior pharyngeal flap pharyngoplasty). A bridge of tissue is thus formed which, together with movement of the lateral walls of the pharynx, enables closure to occur and allows better separation of the oral and nasal cavities. An alternative method is to bulk out the rear wall of the pharynx so that the soft palate does not have such a wide gap to cover in order to produce effective closure. This is usually achieved by stitching two flaps of tissue taken from the lateral pharyngeal wall onto the posterior pharyngeal wall above Passavant's Ridge (Hyne's pharyngoplasty).

Despite intervention in the form of both surgery and therapy it may not always be possible for the cleft palate child to obtain completely normal speech. However, in most cases, speech will eventually be readily intelligible and many cleft palate children do achieve speech which sounds normal to an untrained ear.

In my own clinical work I have occasionally come across adults who had clefts repaired many years ago, when communication therapy was not so readily available as it is nowadays. One lady was in her fifties when I met her and her speech had many typical features. The first repair had been carried out when she was an infant and then in her teens she had what I understood to be a pharyngoplasty. This second surgery improved her nasality to the point where she could produce most consonants clearly in isolation. If asked to say 'd' she could. Sadly she had never been helped to incorporate these new sounds into her established but faulty sound system, so she still persisted in substituting nasals for other consonants, or omitting consonants altogether. If asked to say 'day' she would produce 'ay'. This meant her speech was essentially a string of vowels and very hard to understand. This lady was resistant to any suggestion that she should attempt to change her speech at such a late stage; she had invested much in coping with it as it was. I was saddened by her story because had she received some further help after the pharyngoplasty in her teens, her speech could have been transformed.

By contrast, another lady arrived in my clinic at the ripe age of eighty. She had been spotted by a sensitive doctor and sent along for a chat. When I saw her she was, and always had been, desperately ashamed of her speech. She had never known that anything could be done for people like herself and had never had any therapy. I told her that while her speech couldn't sound normal, it could sound considerably better. She was shocked and excited and insisted on starting work immediately.

5

Dysphasia, dysarthria, and dyspraxia

DYSPHASIA

Dysphasia is a disorder of language, language being the process by which we use symbols to communicate with others and to order our own thoughts. A dysphasic person's use and understanding of symbols is therefore not reliable. Dysphasia is a disorder of symbolism. We receive messages both auditorily through spoken language and visually by writing and gestures. We send messages to other people via the same channels. More often than not these channels are used together as with speech and gesture. It follows that dysphasia can affect any or all of these channels. Although speech is by far the most important and flexible modality within language, there is a great deal more to communicating than speech alone and clinical staff should be wary of assessing for a possible dysphasia simply by listening to the patient's speech. Admittedly speech is the most accessible pointer to the presence or otherwise of dysphasia, but general conversation may not necessarily reflect the client's understanding of language, their reading or writing ability, the use and understanding of gesture, or the use and understanding of non-verbal behaviour. So rather than describing the pathology of a person's speech, we need to think in terms of the overall pathology of their language.

Terminology

Strictly speaking the term asphasia describes a complete inability to use language, in contrast to the less severe dysphasia. More usually they are used interchangeably. Mild, moderate and severe are all used to denote the degree of impairment and so a person may be described as having a severe, moderate or minimal dysphasia. Language is really much too complex to be categorized in this way but these terms are used. In practice it is important to remember that a minimal dysphasia is only minimal in relation to moderate and severe dysphasia. Even a mild impairment can cause enormous problems and is likely to lose someone a job, reduce reading to a chore and take all the pleasure out of social banter. If you had even a minimal language deficit you would be unlikely to be able to read and assimilate this text. Strictly speaking, if the dysphasia has some effect on all the language modalities of spoken and written words, or gesture at any level, then that person is globally aphasic, although global is more commonly used to refer to a severe deficit across all modalities. The most common cause of dysphasia in adults is stroke, others being head injury and brain tumours. (The term dyslexia describes a specific impairment of reading ability which occurs independently of other language deficits and with or without an accompanying writing deficit (dysgraphia).)

Classification

At the simplest level this has long been couched in terms of expressive and receptive problems. Although to a certain extent this can be a straightforward way of thinking about dysphasia, it has limitations as pure disorders of either expressive or receptive ability are very rare. The nature of dysphasia is such that the central meanings and concepts of language become disorganized, thus affecting both understanding and expression to some degree. Classically, dysphasia has been described according to the localization of language function within the dominant cerebral hemisphere (Fig. 5.1). Damage to Wernicke's area (the posterior part

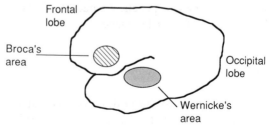

Fig. 5.1 The language areas of the cortex.

of the upper temporal convolution) will produce a dysphasia in which the client produces a lot of fluent nonsense sounds (jargon) which almost sound real because intonation is preserved. Such a client would have severe comprehension problems. Damage to Broca's area (the inferior frontal convolution) will produce a hesitant, groping speech with the most noticeable feature being an inability to find the correct words (anomia or word finding difficulty). Such a person would also be expected to have a comprehension deficit but not necessarily as catastrophic as in the Wernicke type.

It is not abnormal to experience some dysphasic symptoms on a day-to-day basis. Most of us are familiar with losing a word, very commonly someone's name: 'Did I tell you I'd seen Mrs . . . oh what's her name? It's on the tip of my tongue.' Accompanying this word loss there is usually an awareness of the word so that you know it is a name you have encountered before and that if someone offered a name you would recognize whether it was the one you were searching for. You may also have a vague hunch that the word begins with or contains a certain sound. We are more prone to experience such word finding difficulties when we are tired. It is frustrating enough when it occurs as a one-off event in this way, but dysphasic people are likely to struggle many times in the course of one sentence. Migraine sufferers may experience temporary dysphasia alongside visual and sensory disturbances.

ASSESSMENT OF DYSPHASIA

We receive the communications of others via speech, writing and gesture, and produce our own messages in the same way (Fig. 5.2). A full assessment of dysphasia would involve cross-

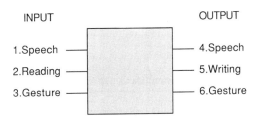

Fig. 5.2 Input and output channels of language.

referencing of all channels, incorporating various levels of complexity and abstraction. By presenting someone with the written word 'apple' and asking them to read it aloud, the link between channels 2 and 4 are being tested albeit at a very elementary level. Presenting the written question 'Which is the odd one out from cat, apple, dog?', and asking for a spoken answer, again tests the links between channels 2 and 4 but at a more complex level (Fig. 5.3). The spoken instruction 'Tell me the steps involved in making a cup of tea,' will involve channel 1 at a fairly elementary level, because the task needs to be understood, but a rather more complex manipulation at channel 4 (Fig. 5.4).

One of the major problems that arises in testing dysphasia stems from the fact that it is extremely difficult to assess the processing of language in the brain without testing the input and output channels at the same time. When attempting to examine receptive skills beyond all but a very basic level, the intrinsic difficulty cannot be avoided that any presented language task not only has to be grasped and understood, but also requires a language based response. Conversely, the assessment of expressive abilities requires that the nature of the task has to be understood. The client has to realize what he is being asked to do. This all makes

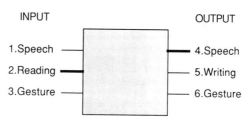

Fig. 5.3 Different language tasks involve the selective use of channels.

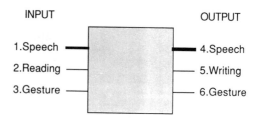

Fig. 5.4 Some tasks place different levels of demand on the respective processes. Here the command itself is not complex but the language skills required to formulate and deliver a response are.

ascertaining the relative contributions of receptive and expressive deficits even more convoluted, nevertheless there are numerous dysphasia assessments on the market and new ones are constantly appearing. Published tests tend to be long and complex and even a popular screening assessment may contain something like a hundred separate items which have to be presented to a client. Common tests in everyday clinical use include the Minnesota Test for the Differential Diagnosis of Aphasia (Schuell, 1965), the Aphasia Screening Test (Whurr, 1974) and the Boston Diagnostic Aphasia Examination (Goodglass and Kaplan, 1983). There are many others for assessing individual features of dysphasia such as the Sentence Comprehension Test (Wheldall, Mittler and Hobsbaum, 1979) and the Graded Naming Test (McKenna and Warrington, 1983).

Most assessments are only reliable when administered by suitably qualified professionals, usually communication therapists, psychologists and sometimes linguists. Some publishers operate a system of restricted access to these publications and maintain a register of qualified users. However, there are now two language screening tests which are quick to administer and have been designed specifically for use by people in other disciplines with no background in language pathology. These are the Frenchay Aphasia Screening Test, FAST (Enderby et al., 1987) which screens for dysphasia and the Sheffield Screening Test for Acquired Language Disorder (Syder et al., in press) which screens for moderate to high level language deficits.

Effect on comprehension

It is often reported that a severely dysphasic person '. . . understands everything that's said, he just can't get his words out'. This is very rarely, if ever true. The misunderstanding arises because even severely verbally impaired clients often retain some awareness of gesture, facial expression and context. However, in the absence of contextual clues these same clients are not able to respond appropriately to even the most elementary verbal message. This is particularly noticeable in a hospital setting where patients become accustomed to a ward routine, making their ability to carry out certain commands an unreliable guide to their understanding of verbal material. A nurse might be certain that her patient has reasonable comprehension because when she

71

instructs him to have a wash he does so. She does not allow for the possibility that he has observed that at certain times of the day particular sequences of activity involve washing. Without realizing it she may even have provided a context for her verbal instruction 'Would you like to have a wash?' by appearing with a bowl of water, soap and a towel. Or it may be that the client is able to pick out key words, in this case the word 'wash' and infer the meaning of the whole sentence from it. His carrying out of the activity indicates a functional ability or how much use he is able to make of the abilities he has, but it does not give a realistic picture of his formal ability to understand language.

The symbolic understanding of severely dysphasic clients may be so reduced that they are not able to deal with symbols even in a rudimentary way. It is common for dysphasic people to be unable to link verbal symbols with the real object. This can be demonstrated by presenting two or three familiar items such as a cup, spoon and pen and asking the client 'Which is the spoon?' If he does not understand what is being asked of him this can be clarified by demonstration or rephrasing the request: 'Show me the spoon.' Point to the spoon.' Invariably clients who are able to grasp what is required will point to one of the objects but they will only pick the right one if they have enough symbolic understanding to link the sound 'spoon' with the real object. The greater the number of choices offered, the harder a dysphasic person will find the task. So someone who can correctly select the spoon from a group of three objects may fail to select it from a group of ten. In some instances of Wernicke type dysphasia, where there is frequently a catastrophic breakdown in symbolic processing, the person may not even be able to link pictures of an object with the real thing, even though the picture is a coloured photograph of an identical object. He cannot see that there is anything to link the symbol and object. The same lack of comprehension of verbal labels will usually apply to written as well as spoken words so that if the same client is handed a piece of paper with the word 'spoon' written clearly on it, he cannot place it with the spoon and may instead put it with the cup or another object. Occasionally the actual presentation of the symbol has some bearing on whether the client can understand it and he may have a better comprehension of upper-case rather than lower-case letters. Frequently dysphasic clients are able to process printed words more easily than those written in longhand.

At a less severe level of impairment, dysphasic clients are able to understand the general gist of a conversation when the conditions under which the conversation takes place are favourable, e.g. there is no background noise and the client is not tired or anxious. This will only hold true if the conversation centres around topics of particular interest for the client and when the inclusion of complex grammatical constructions and abstract concepts is kept to a minimum.

The same applies to reading and so clients may well be able to follow straightforward written sentences on concrete topics and interpret a variety of written messages in everyday use (bus destinations, names of shops, etc.) but still be baffled by a full newspaper article and a subtle turn of phrase. Such a person can deal with the mechanics of reading but miss the nuances of understanding that are necessary for following and enjoying the plot of a novel. They frequently remark that though they can still read, they don't enjoy it as much as they used to because it is time consuming and hard work. They may attribute this to lack of concentration but in fact reading now requires extra concentration and effort as it is no longer automatic.

The dysphasic client with mild receptive problems can easily miss being diagnosed by clinicians. While the client may appear to understand it may need a tremendous effort of concentration to sustain this and not be 'caught out'. They will have to concentrate hard on various activities such as reading the paper, watching television or talking with friends, all of which were previously dealt with effortlessly.

Effect on expression

Expressive language is used in many forms ranging from propounding a detailed abstract theory to writing a shopping list, from answering a simple question to writing an essay, from shrugging the shoulders to elegant pantomime.

A client whose expressive language is severely dysphasic may be limited to a repeated word, syllable or phrase in spontaneous speech. 'Yes' and 'No' responses can be unreliable and may conflict with the simultaneous non-verbal message, so that the person nods their head at the same time as saying 'No'. Although he may be able to complete simple cued phrases such as 'Give me the knife and . . .', and perhaps count to ten or recite parts of the alphabet when helped, he is unlikely to be able to put even these minimal abilities to any functional use. He may not be able to write his own name and although many dysphasics do retain some awareness of the meaning of gestures they seem unable to use gesture extensively to supplement their communication. The ability to swear fluently is often retained either as an automatic response or as a result of emotional disinhibition and while this may serve to relieve the client's frustration it does cause great embarrassment for friends and relatives. This is more likely to be the case in Wernicke's aphasia where usually the client is not aware that he is swearing and is mortified if made aware of it.

WERNICKE'S APHASIA (FLUENT APHASIA)

The fluent pattern consists of what is sometimes called a 'word salad' or jargon. Here, although speech retains some elements of grammatical structure, overall output is nonsensical. There may be substitutions of sounds so that 'pable' is used instead of 'table', or words so that 'chair' is used instead of 'table'. This sentence was written by a fluent dysphasic patient asked to write a sentence which included the word 'hospital':

Infectious diseases reduce in Sheffield holidays.

The client typically shows very little ability to monitor their own output, paralleled by poor understanding of the speech of others. The speech may include many completely non-English words, this type of expressive language being known as jargon aphasia. Writing may follow a similar pattern, namely retained access to language but poor control over its production and lack of inhibition of incorrect uses. Figure 5.5 shows the responses of Bill (a 60-year-old man with a severe jargon dysphasia after a stroke), on a writing task. He was presented with the spoken instruction 'Write your name'. The comprehension difficulty has led to his misinterpreting the request and writing my name instead. He has picked out the key words 'write' and 'name' but ignored the other necessary grammatical information. When the command was repeated 'Write YOUR name', the second attempt was correct (Fig. 5.5).

Bill was then asked to respond in writing to the question 'Where are we now?' Note the incorrect sequencing of the words (Fig. 5.6). He was aiming for Royal Hallamshire Hospital and we can see his partial success. People familiar with Bill's lifestyle might

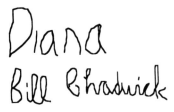

Fig. 5.5 The written response of Bill, a severe jargon dysphasic to the spoken instruction 'Write your name'.

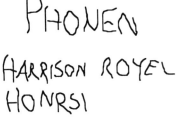

Fig. 5.6 The response of the same man asked to respond in writing to the query 'Where are we now?'

be able to guess his intent from the written clues he has been able to give.

The initial error in Fig. 5.5 was brought to Bill's attention and his drawing of me in Fig. 5.7 is his attempt to acknowledge the nature of the error. Bill, rather unusually, spontaneously used drawing to supplement his communication and later extended this use of visual symbols to include painting as a means of self-expression.

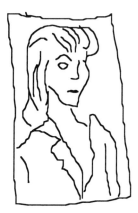

Fig. 5.7 Bill acknowledges his first error by drawing the therapist.

BROCA'S APHASIA (NON-FLUENT)

Non-fluent output is characterized by a hesitant telegrammatic style of speech and writing. Telegrammatic refers to the use of language occasioned when it is necessary to include only the absolutely vital elements of a linguistic structure. 'Arrive 9 a.m. main station' is a telegrammatic message and is the sort of thing that might actually be written on a telegram, where the economy of language also results in the saving of money. Just enough of the full sentence is retained to convey meaning and avoid ambiguity. Non-fluent dysphasic clients appear to search for the important words and omit the smaller grammatical words which hold sentences together. 'Tea . . . hot . . . milk', is a typical non-fluent sentence. The general topic and meaning is conveyed but there is much ambiguity. Here are some extracts from the diary of Arthur, a dysphasic man. They are presented exactly as written.

8 July
CHURCH if BREAKFAST. MORNING SERVICE
   (WITH COMMUNION).
Women's Fellowship in the lounge.
We for the Flower Festival.
Be to GRAVES about. the still back
you sunny. I was both enjoyed to the full. animals and leaved
   you
became come about.
Graves about MOTOR. about
the AIRWAYS remains. unders.

10 July
I this in Cleethorpe as time
drawrin upto, another prenen one sec
good new cosr that beech
We asked to beat expernape, with certainly
other who have deal.
How fortunate such teathers are.
They canot only non, stop from now
only non- stop now
They can ask themselves all the right
as WELL.

12 July
You owe so much to yourself you cannot
afford owe anybody else
Dishonesty is never an accident.
Good men like good women never see temptation when they
  meet it.
Don't go anything here which hurts
your self-respect.
Don't tell me what I'd like to hear
but what I ought to hear. I don't
want a valet to my vanity.

21 July
A Hero holidaymaker from Sheffield
strong seas to save drowning
swimmer in a seaside rescue – then
quietly. to avoid glory. a man
floundering 100 yards out to sea.
He across the water to reach bather
in trouble off the old Skegness Pier
– and him to the shore –.

In the first two entries the language retains some recognizable
structure and although it is impossible to obtain an accurate meaning from it, nevertheless we can gain some sense of what has been
happening. There are some inversions of word order but on the
whole the sequencing of words remains grammatically correct. In
the excerpt for the 12th July, Arthur has copied certain aphorisms
that appealed to him from another text. In the last section for the
21st July, he has obviously copied sections out of a newspaper
account of events in order to record the information. This is a
strategy commonly adopted by non-fluent dysphasics in their writing. Note the inconsistent use of upper- and lower-case script and
the layout of the lines on the page.

REHABILITATION OF THE DYSPHASIC PERSON

Once the client is medically stable the rehabilitation of communication is the responsibility of a communication therapist.

1. *Direct intervention* involves input by the therapist directly with the clients;
2. *Indirect intervention* involves work by the therapist with those in the client's environment.

Direct intervention

Some direct therapy attempts to influence the client's actual language ability by facilitating and restoring discrete skills. Such skills include perceiving one sound as different from another (auditory discrimination), being able to pick out particular words in a passage (auditory attention) and the recall of vocabulary or naming and using symbols in one modality to link up with those in another to facilitate their understanding and production (e.g. word/picture matching). There are many more techniques that have been devised to isolate and practise the individual skills required for language which are used as part of an overall programme of rehabilitation. Other direct therapy concentrates on how the client uses a particular skill once he has command of it. Being able to say the word 'table' does not necessarily mean the word will be used appropriately when it is needed. Similarly at a more complex level, knowing the forms of various greetings does not automatically mean they will be used at the right time with the right people. Some work on adapting the client's social skills to fit his new circumstances is often necessary to help him make the most of his abilities.

Counselling the client constitutes another form of direct intervention. Language is such a complex and important part of our lives that most people are not automatically equipped to make the drastic transition from coping with themselves as a communicator to coping with themselves as a non-communicator. Many dysphasics and their relatives find themselves in a state of utter bewilderment at the onset of dysphasia, often followed by feelings of helplessness and withdrawal (Chapter 9).

Direct therapy also encourages people to supplement damaged speech with a combination of whatever channels are available to them, including writing, gesture and drawing. They are often resistant to do this as they perceive such an approach to be tantamount to giving up on oral communication and second best. This is partly due to a lack of understanding of just how much other modalities normally contribute to our daily communication and partly because clients are unable to accept that speech will not eventually return. Sadly, the failure to incorporate other modalities results in the communication being less successful than it might otherwise be and inevitably leads to isolation.

Indirect intervention

Carers may be required to carry out specific linguistic activities or assignments at home as part of an overall programme where there is only periodic contact with a therapist.

Indirect therapy may also use explanation, advice and counselling of the immediate family and others in the client's environment in order to adapt that environment so as to make the best functional use of the person's residual abilities. It would also pay attention to helping those in close relationships with the client to come to terms, as far as possible, with what has happened.

IS THERAPY SUCCESSFUL?

Basically it depends what criteria are used to define success. This is a contentious question, the answer to which is the subject of much ongoing research and evaluation. It is indisputable that counselling and environmental work are effective in re-introducing some quality of life for the client. As in most disciplines, both successes and failures are reported for the more empirical therapies.

One of the difficulties in investigating dysphasia treatment arises from the assumption that the disorder falls into neat categories and as we have already seen this is not the case. In addition, the subtle differences of personality, motivation and pre-morbid linguistic ability between individuals often make assessment of one particular therapy across a group of patients unreliable because it is so hard to control for such a large number of variables. Until now, evaluation of direct language therapy has consisted of comparing treatment and no-treatment control groups but without standardizing the therapeutic approaches used.

An alternative research strategy that avoids some of the problems mentioned above, but which tends to be seen as inferior scientific method, uses single case studies. A patient is treated intensively for one aspect of the deficit, which, if the therapy is successful, might be expected to improve disproportionately to other accompanying deficits.

At the moment results of the various investigations are often contradictory, but as techniques both for administering and evaluating language therapy become more sophisticated, it seems likely that a situation will emerge where certain types of language impairment are shown to be directly amenable to specific therapeutic strategies, whereas others will be shown to be less so.

Either way the involvement of a therapist with a client is long term. Most spontaneous recovery is seen in the first few months after onset of dysphasia as in the dysphasia after stroke, but substantial improvements in language ability can be expected for up to one year (Fig. 5.8). This is not to say that there will be no further change in the client's functional communication skills after this time. On the contrary, social and emotional adjustments mean that communication can improve for several years post-trauma.

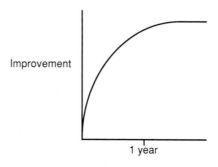

Fig. 5.8 Language recovery after a stroke.

STRATEGIES TO IMPROVE COMMUNICATION WITH A DYSPHASIC PERSON

Having a conversation with someone who is even minimally dysphasic can be very hard work. By modifying your own output it is possible to help them perform at maximum linguistic and functional potential. The following strategies help:

1. Cut down on outside distractions.
A dysphasic person is less able to ignore another conversation

going on in the same room, the sound of a hairdryer or people walking past. In a hospital ward it helps to draw the bed curtains to cut out visual distractions and to turn off televisions and radios.

2. Speak slowly.
Slowing the rate of speech will give more time for material to be processed, but it is important to retain normal rhythm and intonation. The dysphasic person needs time both to take in what you have said and to answer. This is probably the single most important measure you can take. A dysphasic person will communicate best when relaxed. If they try too hard, speech will suffer.

3. Use simple and concrete language but don't talk down to the client.
Because a dysphasic tends to rely on literal messages they find it hard to interpret humour and sarcasm, which can lead to distress.

4. Don't change topics quickly.
A dysphasic person needs extra time to tune in to the topic of a conversation. For this reason:

a. avoid group conversations wherever possible.
b. use a verbal lead in – 'I meant to ask you . . .'
                            'By the way . . .'
                            'Let's talk about . . .'
c. try to convey only one idea at a time.
d. use short sentences.
e. establish a context so the person knows what you are referring to, e.g. 'I want to talk about your holiday.'

5. Pause between phrases.
This allows each item to sink in;
e.g. 'Your glasses . . . are in the cupboard . . . by the bed.'

6. Use less ambiguous phrases.
Specify exactly what, where, when and who you are talking about, e.g. 'I'll put the tablets in *the cupboard*, rather than, 'I'll put them over here'.

7. Don't shout.
If you suspect a hearing loss a hearing test should be arranged. Raising the volume of your voice does not improve comprehension. If anything it will make things worse as shouting distorts normal intonation, stress patterns and lip movements, all of which are used as clues by the dysphasic person.

8. Check that the client understands you.
You may need to:

a. ask the person to recount your message if their expressive ability allows this.
b. repeat your message in different ways rather than repeating exactly the same words over and over again.

    e.g. 'What's your address?'
        'Where do you live?'
        'Where are you from?'
        'What's the name of your street?'
        'Where's home?'

This takes practice, but becomes easier.

c. be careful not to mistake alertness for understanding. Dysphasia is very distressing and embarrassing and people often try to hide their difficulties. As a rough guide, if there is *any* language deficit that is detectable in everyday expression, then there will be comprehension problems as well.

9. Check that you understand the client.
You may need to:

a. stop the conversation as soon as you do not understand in order to make backtracking easier.
b. supplement spoken 'yes' and 'no' with nodding, shaking the head or thumbs up and down to avoid confusion.
c. watch facial expressions for clues.
d. if the client is having great difficulty in expressing a particular idea, leave the topic and move to something else; the sought after words will often slip out when the person is distracted.

10. Encourage the client:

a. to use other modalities – writing, drawing, gesture.
b. to make an attempt to communicate. Do not criticize however incomplete or incorrect the attempt may be.
c. to take some responsibility for the conversation, e.g. if you have to leave a conversation because you simply cannot understand, try to do so by mutual consent. The client has then participated in the decision as to how to handle the difficulty.

You can do this by asking 'Is it important?' or 'Can we leave it for the time being?'

11.   Don't pretend you understand.
The client will eventually realize what you are doing and conclude that you are not interested in what they are saying. In addition, the client themselves may not realize that the conversation has gone astray and therefore cannot begin to attempt any correction until it is brought to his attention.

12.   Include the client in conversations.
Encourage other people to take time to converse with the patient and not to ignore him. Even if the client finds it hard to make any response at all you can still use eye-contact to involve him in the interaction.

13.   Don't expect too much of yourself.
Talking to someone with dysphasia is not easy, no matter how hard you both work at it or how many 'rules' you follow. It is an intrinsically frustrating and difficult situation. Don't be too disappointed if you can't understand everything the client is trying to say, or if you cannot get all your own messages across. The important thing is to keep trying so the person does not experience social isolation and human contact at some level is maintained.

DYSARTHRIA

Normal speech production depends on the functioning of the following muscles together with their nerve supply:

1.   Abdominal muscles and diaphragm;
2.   Intercostal muscles;
3.   Laryngeal structures;
4.   Muscles of the mid-pharynx and posterior tongue that shape the pharyngeal cavity;
5.   Palatopharyngeal muscles;
6.   Middle and anterior tongue muscles;
7.   Facial muscles used in protruding, retracting, opening and closing the lips;
8.   Muscles that work the mandible.

Impairment of any of these may result in slurred speech or dysarthria by changing:

1. strength of muscle contraction;
2. speed of movement;
3. range of movement;
4. accuracy of movement;
5. steadiness of movement;
6. muscle tone.

Different types of dysarthria will result in different clusters of symptoms depending on which part of the neuromuscular system is affected. There are various ways of classifying these types, the most commonly encountered is probably that based on the site of the lesion. This may be in the peripheral muscles, lower motor neurones, upper motor neurones, extra-pyramidal system, cerebellum and its connections or in the cerebral cortex.

The umbrella term of dysarthria incorporates many specific deficits.

DYSARTHRIC SYMPTOMS

The processes of respiration, phonation, resonance and articulation are all involved in the mechanical production of normal speech and so although dysarthria is considered to be a disorder of articulation, deficits in any one of these processes will serve to reduce intelligibility.

Respiration

Good lung capacity maintains an adequate volume and enables speech to be phrased in an appropriate way. More control is needed when breathing for speech than in quiet respiration, and normal speech only occurs on expiration. Quiet expiration is a passive process with the rib cage returning to its uninflated rest position as a result of the elastic recoil of the lungs. Expiration during speech however is an active process with the intercostal muscles slowing the rate of descent of the rib cage.

Poor control of inspiration and expiration will interfere with stress and intonation patterns, both of which play an important part in determining the intelligibility of speech. Many dysarthrics have distorted stress and intonation.

Phonation

Paresis of the vocal cords will result in a weak and breathy sounding voice which tires easily. Volume will tail off after periods of talking or towards the end of sentences. Lack of vocal cord control interferes with the pitch mechanism and therefore intonation (Chapter 6). The overall pitch may drop or be raised, speech may be monotonous and inexpressive. Intonation patterns are vital for the effortless understanding of speech by the listener and without good control it becomes impossible for the speaker to portray subtle shades of meaning. Accurate initiation of phonation is vital for distinguishing between voiced, e.g. /b/d/g/z/ and voiceless sounds, e.g. /p/t/k/s/, etc.

Resonance

The soft palate and pharynx together act as a valve which directs the airstream either through the nose or the mouth. Wherever there is palatal insufficiency, voice quality either has too little resonance (hyponasality) or too much resonance (hypernasality) and there is the same difficulty in making oral and nasal contrasts as we find in cleft palate speech.

Articulation

Neuromuscular impairment of the moveable articulators (tongue, lips, soft palate, lower jaw) produces slurred speech as the tongue and lips cannot change the shape of the intra-oral cavity sufficiently to differentiate between vowels or consonants. Precise consonant production involves close contact or approximation between one or more of the articulators and some other part of the intra-oral space. Normal articulation involves very rapid and accurate movement of the articulators and if they cannot move quickly enough and are therefore pulled away to form the next sound before adequate contact has been made, the movement is left incomplete and the sound is indistinct. If the deficit is severe the muscles may be incapable of making the contact at all. The articulation deficit may vary from slight slurring to a complete inability to produce differentiated sounds where speech is reduced to unrecognizable grunts.

ASSESSMENT OF DYSARTHRIA

Structured subjective tests such as the Frenchay Dysarthria Assessment (Enderby, 1983) and the Robertson Dysarthria Profile (Robertson, 1982) enable a comprehensive description to be made of a dysarthric person's speech. These are useful for analysing which features of the dysarthria are contributing most significantly to the impaired intelligibility and in indicating priority areas for remediation. Some features of the speech can be measured objectively. A measure of palatal competence can be gained by assessing the emission of air through the nose using a nasal anemometer or by videofluoroscopy where an X-ray picture shows the movement of the soft palate and pharynx. Voice pitch and frequency can be displayed and measured on computers.

REHABILITATION OF THE DYSARTHRIC PERSON

The dysarthric client has to learn to adjust and compensate for the loss of automatic, easy speech. The mechanical production of speech becomes a great effort and the more concrete aim of being

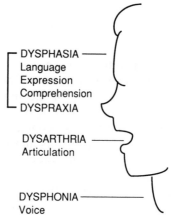

DYSPHASIA ——
Language
Expression
Comprehension
DYSPRAXIA

DYSARTHRIA ——
Articulation

DYSPHONIA ————
Voice

Fig. 5.9 Speech and language breakdown.

understood now has to take precedence over that of individual and effective expression. He must learn continuously to monitor and correct his own speech output and can no longer rely on built in feedback systems to do this for him. He has to concentrate on exactly how he is saying things, as well as on what he is saying. This continual concentration is tiring and many people cannot sustain it throughout conversation. The client now has voluntarily to coordinate his articulators, breath supply and phonation, yet despite great effort may only achieve a very poor control of speech.

The management of dysarthria concentrates on increasing self-monitoring and voluntary control of the impaired systems. Initially the client's speech needs to be thoroughly assessed to gauge the relative functioning of all the component systems as well as the overall intelligibility of speech. Direct work may be done on difficult sounds or groups of sounds, slowing the rate of speech, volume control, pitch control, breathing, phrasing and intonation. Consideration has to be given to what will make the speech socially acceptable, not just to what will make it clearer. Even if a dysarthric person has intelligible speech which is produced at an unacceptably loud volume, people will be uncomfortable in their company.

Dysarthrics often achieve markedly improved intelligibility in speech clinics where concentration is easier and where a therapist's monitoring supplements the patient's own awareness. However, generalizing this to less structured situations outside the clinic is often difficult because we are accustomed to giving the whole of our attention to the content of a conversation rather than to the mechanics of it. To compound the difficulty, conversations usually move more quickly outside a speech clinic and it is impossible for a dysarthric person to regain the speed necessary for any degree of spontaneity. In an effort to keep up and stay involved, the person invariably sacrifices his self-monitoring and the bulk of the responsibility for the conversation is shifted onto the listener, who is then expected to interpret whatever sounds are being produced. When the dysarthria is part of a progressive disorder such as motor neurone disease or multiple sclerosis some clients can benefit from therapy to boost their speech awareness and increase motivation.

IMPROVING COMMUNICATION WITH A DYSARTHRIC PERSON

1. Check for understanding.

If you do not understand what has been said, say so and ask for a repetition. It doesn't matter if you have to do this several times over the same section of speech. Even more so than in dysphasia, clients will be quick to recognize any faking of understanding. They usually do not object to repeating themselves. If you make these checks as soon as you start to lose the thread there will be less back-tracking to do. You can save time in a longer sentence by repeating those parts you do understand as shown in the example, otherwise you may have to sit through a second version of what may be a long account.

> *client:* We took my niece and nephew to the circus last Friday. It was their first time and they were really excited. Lisa was thrilled by the jugglers.
> *therapist:* You took your niece and nephew to the circus last Friday . . . and then what?'
> or
> *client:* I went to see Mrs Sanders at two o'clock.
> *therapist:* You went to see who at two o'clock?

2. Help monitor the speech.

Most dysarthric people can adjust the clarity of their speech to some extent if you simply remind them to '. . . slow down and make it clearer'.

3. Watch turn-taking.

Pay attention to facial expression and other cues so you are aware when your conversational partner is wanting to take up a turn. Leave longer pauses so he can initiate his turn comfortably without having to compete with you. Make sure you give him time to complete his turn. Occasionally dysarthrics learn to over-compensate for their diminished roles in conversations by using various strategies that enable them to hang on to their own turns far too long. With these people you will feel that *you* can't get a word in edgeways. In this case you are allowed to assert your own rights in the conversation and interrupt. If interruption doesn't work, it might be worth bringing this to their notice.

4. Make sure you can receive non-verbal cues.

Have a clear view of their face and mouth so you can take advantage of facial expression and use lip-reading to supplement your comprehension.

5. Cut down on distractions.
Particularly auditory ones. This enables both of you to concentrate and gives you a better chance of picking up those sounds they manage to produce.

6. Use other modalities.
Don't be afraid to produce paper and pen, especially to clarify key words such as names.

7. Give feedback.
The dysarthric person will be slow in getting through his sentences especially if the dysarthria is severe. He will be only too aware of this and needs reassurance that you are still attending. The usual nodding, 'mmm' and eye-contact will suffice.

DYSPRAXIA

Lesions causing dyspraxia usually involve the post-central area of the parietal lobe, though the temporal lobe is sometimes implicated. This is an impairment of the ability to perform purposeful and voluntary movements despite the fact that the relevant neuro-muscular systems are intact. This means a movement can be made automatically but not voluntarily. Dyspraxia can affect any voluntary motor movement but when speech is affected it is termed articulatory dyspraxia, verbal dyspraxia or dyspraxia of speech. The speaker knows the word he wants to say but cannot coordinate the necessary muscle movements into the right sequences to make the correct sounds. Hence a dyspraxic person may greet you with a wide smile, but be quite unable to imitate that same movement when asked. At a more complex level they may say 'Hello' as a greeting but be unable to repeat it when requested to 'Say that again' or 'Say hello.' Similarly they will be able to lick their lips and chew whilst eating, but not in imitation of another person. Automatic speech such as counting or reciting the days of the week may be intact but the same words are not accessible for correct use in a different context. Someone with a less severe dyspraxia will experience difficulty only with polysyllabic words or the more complex sound combinations and may be able to perform certain manoeuvres at a slow rate, but not as they attempt to speed up to a normal rate of speech. In some ways dyspraxia can seem a more bizarre condition than either dysarthria or dysphasia.

A dyspraxic person can characteristically be seen groping for the correct sequencing of articulatory movements as they try out a number of possibilities in the hope of hitting the right one. While engaged in this trial and error approach, their lips and tongue will move in a contorted and laboured fashion. Although dyspraxia is frequently accompanied by some degree of dysphasia, language abilities can be comparatively intact and levels of awareness and hence frustration are very high. The person embarks on a particular sound and something quite different and unintended comes out, a condition that is extremely difficult both for them and their family to understand.

ASSESSMENT OF DYSPRAXIA

The most commonly used formal clinical assessments ask the client to say groups of sounds and words of increasing complexity. In this way the type and level of errors can be analysed and a comprehensive picture formed of the nature and extent of the dyspraxia. The Apraxia Battery for Adults (Dabul, 1979) and the Test for Oral Dyspraxia (Darley *et al.*, 1975) are tests of this type in common clinical use.

REHABILITATION FOR THE DYSPRAXIC PERSON

Once the lesion is physically stable dyspraxia is very resistant to remediation. Rehabilitation techniques aim to improve the position sense of the articulators and oral awareness so the client has more idea of what is happening in his own mouth. They may employ other feedback modalities such as watching oral positions in a mirror and using repetitive vowel and consonant drills to re-establish correct movement patterns. The main push of rehabilitation is aimed at maximizing whatever control is left and supplementing speech with either signs or written systems if necessary.

6

Voice disorders

Any voice which does not have a normal quality is said to be dysphonic. The term aphonia refers to a complete loss of voice, and an aphonic person may either whisper or simply appear to be mouthing the words. Dysphonia is quite different from dysphasia, dysarthria or dyspraxia as it does not interfere with language.

NORMAL VOICE

The following systems must be intact for the production of normal voice:

Energy source   –   Expiration provides a moving column of air.

Sound source   –   The vocal cords adduct and their edges vibrate as the air is forced through.

Resonating system   –   This consists of the nasal and vocal tracts above the level of the cords. The size, shape and tension of the vocal tract modifies and amplifies the fundamental frequencies produced at the larynx, resulting in a voice that is unique for each individual.

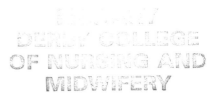

Characteristics of normal voice

1. The voice is easy to listen to and does not sound breathy, hoarse or rough;
2. There is a balance between oral and nasal resonance, i.e. the person does not constantly sound nasal or as if they have a cold;
3. The person uses appropriate volume for the situation;
4. Pitch levels are appropriate for age, sex and size;
5. The voice is expressive and makes use of a range of intonation patterns so that it does not sound monotonous.

An ENT and/or communication therapy referral is needed if:

- the voice frequently sounds gruff, croaky, hoarse or breathy;
- the person habitually uses a voice which is too loud or too quiet;
- the pitch is too high or too low;
- there are frequent episodes of voice loss in the absence of respiratory infections;
- if a child habitually sounds as though he/she has a cold in the absence of other symptoms.

CLASSIFICATION OF VOICE DISORDERS

It is not always easy to classify voice disorders and very often the presenting symptoms will be mixed. There are many links between the traditional divisions of organic, functional and psychogenic voice disorders as long-term psychogenic and functional problems can result in organic changes and functional disorders may involve psychological factors. An example of the latter would be the woman who constantly speaks at a higher pitch than is healthy for her vocal tract because she needs to relate to others as a very 'feminine' woman. The following is a guide to how voice disorders are classified.

Organic

Congenital:　　　　　　laryngeal web, cleft palate, laryngo-malacia.

Tumours:	malignant and benign.
Trauma:	intubation granulomas.
Neurological:	vocal cord palsies, spastic dysphonia (see also psychogenic disorders below).
Endocrine disorders:	myxodoema, hyperthyroidism.
Inflammatory:	laryngitis.

Functional

These disorders are caused by factors directly attributable to the vocal *habits* of a person and would not otherwise develop. They include

vocal nodules (singer's nodes)
contact ulcers
vocal strain

Psychogenic

Here there is no obvious pathology either organic or functional.

conversion (hysterical) aphonia/dysphonia
puberphonia
mutism
spastic dysphonia (see also organic disorders)

Iatrogenic

The symptoms are induced by the actions of the clinician, e.g. cord palsy following cardiac or thoracic surgery.

ORGANIC VOICE DISORDERS

Congenital voice problems

Congenital abnormalities of the larynx (glottis) are generally detected soon after birth and treated surgically. Supraglottic and glottic obstructions in the infant produce obvious phonation on

93

inspiration, as in laryngomalacia where the supraglottic tissues are lax and collapse on inspiration. Subglottic stenosis and subglottic haemangioma cause stridor on both inspiration and expiration.

In some infants allergies and prolonged upper respiratory tract infections, or exposure to irritants such as smoke, can be the cause of harsh sounding voices.

Voice problems as a result of abuse and/or misuse (see later) are rare in a healthy infant but some congenital conditions such as Down's Syndrome may predispose a child to vocal behaviours which cause cord damage later on.

Tumours

Malignant lesions

Of laryngeal tumours 95% are malignant. Supraglottic tumours account for 40–45%, glottic tumours for 50–55% and subglottic tumours for 5% of these. Different symptoms are likely to present first in the different types and cord lesions give rise to hoarseness earlier in their history than lesions in other laryngeal sites. They are also more likely to be well differentiated and hence patients with glottic tumours have a better prognosis than those with tumours elsewhere in the larynx.

Sixty-five to seventy per cent of detected tumours are in the early stages of their course and are preferably treated using deep X-ray treatment. Complications of radiotherapy include hardening of skin tissue, swallowing problems and sore throats. Surgery is considered in more advanced cases and the glottis is removed in the surgical procedure of laryngectomy. Here the trachea is brought to the neck surface at the level of the excised larynx to form a permanent fistula. This forms the new airway and there is no longer any connection between the trachea and the oral and nasal tracts (Fig. 6.1). The first line of treatment is to help the client to find an alternative sound source which can compensate for the lost larynx. Three methods are commonly employed:

a.   Oesophageal voice
Here the person is taught how to use the top of the oesophagus (at the level of the crico-pharyngeal sphincter), to store small amounts of air and to expel these at will with simultaneous vibration of the oesophageal wall. This sets the air column in the

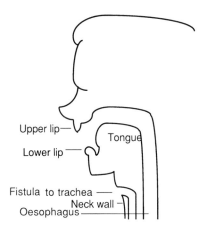

Fig. 6.1 Anatomy of the neck after laryngectomy. The trachea and oesophagus are now separate.

neck vibrating and mouthing words over this airstream will produce recognizable sounds and words. The quality of the sound is characteristically harsh, gravelly and deep in pitch. The person can be understood but is unable to introduce intonation into the speech which is therefore flat and monotonous. In addition there may be the accompanying noise of air being pushed up from the lungs and out through the stoma as the neck muscles contract with the effort of sound production, particularly if the client is trying too hard.

Good oesophageal voice is hard to obtain if there is much scar tissue following the primary surgery, if there has been extensive radiotherapy, or if the patient is bronchitic or suffers from severe respiratory tract infections. Some people find the harsh sound of oesophageal speech unacceptable and are reluctant to use it.

b.   Valve voice
The main difficulty in producing good speech using the oesophageal method is getting enough air into the oesophagus to provide a viable airstream. The last few years have seen the introduction and increasing use of valves to maintain a tracheo-oesophageal fistula, such as the Blom-Singer and Groningen valves. These one-way valves enable the patient to direct air from the trachea into the oesophagus, but they prevent food and drink from passing in the reverse direction. The sound making process

is in effect the same as in oesophageal speech, the difference being in the way the breath supply is maintained (Fig. 6.2).

Valves can either be inserted as part of the primary laryngectomy operation or as a secondary procedure. Not all people are suitable candidates but for those who are the effect on speech can be remarkable. There can be a much more pleasing voice quality and, because airflow is not such a problem, more syllables can be made on one breath and speech is smoother, easier to produce and hence easier to listen to.

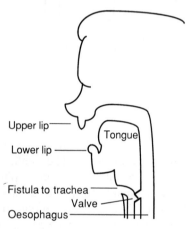

Upper lip

Tongue

Lower lip

Fistula to trachea

Valve

Oesophagus

Fig. 6.2 Anatomy of the neck after laryngectomy and valve insertion. There is a one-way connection between the trachea and oesophagus.

c. Artificial larynx

An artificial sound source can be used as a supplement or replacement for oesophageal voice. There are various models on the market. They consist of a battery driven vibrating disc which is activated by pressing a button on the side of the artificial larynx. When the head is placed against the outside of the neck the vibration is transmitted through the neck tissue and the air in the vocal tract vibrates. When words are mouthed over this they are realized in a mechanical way with a sound similar to that of a speech synthesizer.

There is no intonation in such speech although the overall pitch of the sound can be adjusted to accommodate male and female voices. Some people do achieve very relaxed easy speech with an artificial larynx, and may use it in preference to oesophageal methods or in situations where oesophageal speech is not so effective, such as when talking for long periods or against background noise. One man who used an artificial larynx told of regularly being mistaken for an answering machine when he answered the telephone! Nevertheless he was able to continue his work as a lecturer which he would not have been able to do using oeso-phageal speech alone. Although it takes some practice to become fluent using an artificial larynx many clients are given one to use in the early stages after surgery while they are learning other methods.

Whichever combination of the above rehabilitation approaches works best, laryngectomees have to adapt the way they speak in order to be easily intelligible. They need to slow the rate of speech considerably, adjust phrasing to suit the available air capacity, and exaggerate the mouthing of words in order to make conson-ants clear. Speech will inevitably require more effort than before.

Benign lesions

These are mainly due to inflammatory conditions. Usually acute inflammatory conditions are caused by a general upper respiratory tract infection which is accompanied by a sore throat and red and swollen vocal cords. If there is continued exposure to irritants at this stage such as nicotine, dry or dusty atmospheres, or alcohol, then the laryngitis will persist and become chronic. The healing process will cause changes in the laryngeal tissues and these may be generalized such as granulation and scarring, or localized as with cysts, polyps, nodules and contact ulcers.

Trauma

The laryngeal muscles, cartilages and nerve supply can all be damaged by external trauma. The immediate problem may be airway obstruction and this can require a tracheostomy. If the injuries sustained are so great that the person needs artificial ventilation for some considerable time, the cords can sometimes be damaged by intubation causing intubation granulomas, although such damage is usually avoided by performing a tempo-rary tracheostomy.

Nowadays laser surgery minimizes any scarring that might occur after surgery on the cords themselves such as stripping or the removal of benign lesions and post-operative voice quality is consequently better.

Neurological lesions

Lesions involving the recurrent laryngeal nerve will result in a cord palsy. The left recurrent laryngeal nerve is more vulnerable than its right counterpart as it has a physically longer course, dipping into the chest before rising again into the neck. Hence in thoracic surgery and in procedures which give access the thyroid gland, the left recurrent laryngeal nerve is sometimes damaged, producing a cord palsy. The site of the lesion will determine the position taken up by the affected cord but if it rests near to the midline there may be only a minimal change in voice quality because the non-affected cord can still affect closure and hence produce a vibrating column of air (Fig. 6.3a). If the cord takes up a position away from the midline and the gap is too big for closure to occur the voice will be breathy and there will not be enough breath for normal sentence length as so much air is wasted. Speaking will be an effort and there will be a reduction in volume.

In some cases the normal cord can be strengthened with voice exercises so that it crosses the midline to achieve an off-centre closure. Voice quality in this case may be reasonable. Sometimes it is necessary to bulk out the affected cord with an inert substance such as Teflon, in order to give the good cord something more substantial to vibrate against (Fig. 6.3b)

If despite these manoeuvres the voice remains inadequate, any existing sound can be augmented with hand-held amplifiers.

Endocrine disorders

In myxedema or hypofunction of the thyroid gland voice quality becomes hoarse. This can be treated along with the other symptoms of this condition by giving thyroxine.

Inflammatory disorders

Inflammatory reactions of the vocal folds and surrounding tissues can cause dysphonia. Hoarseness, coughing and sore throats indicate acute laryngitis caused by bacteria, viruses or chemical irritants. Typically, acute laryngitis forms part of a generalized upper respiratory tract infection. In chronic laryngitis the initial cause

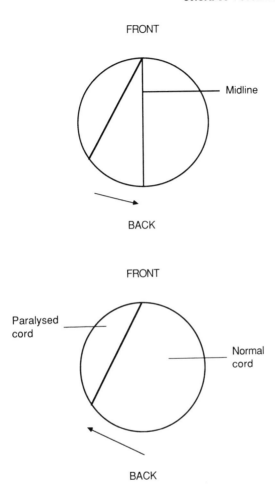

Fig. 6.3 (a) Unilateral vocal cord paralysis. When the cord is fixed at the midline the normal cord can easily achieve closure; (b) when the paralysed cord is fixed away from the midline the normal cord must cross the midline to achieve closure.

of the reaction persists while the healing response results in the formation of granulomas and scar tissue. It is believed that smoking, vocal abuse, dirty atmospheres and alcohol are contributing factors. Chronic laryngitis must be treated and monitored as there can be changes in the epithelial cells resulting in white patches on the cords where excess keratin is being produced. This may indicate the early development of a cancer.

FUNCTIONAL VOICE DISORDERS

Symptoms may result either from a primary disease process or trauma, or from misuse/abuse of the voice which then produces some pathological change.

Vocal abuse and misuse

During phonation the two closing edges of the cords are subject to wear and tear. Vocal abuse refers to such things as excessive shouting, screaming, throat clearing and coughing as well as simply having an excessive talking load. The voice will be harsh in quality, possibly deeper in pitch and have poor volume control. It deteriorates during episodes of use. Vocal misuse includes long-term habitual and inappropriate use of pitch and volume.

For the majority of cases of vocal abuse and misuse the initial stages of successful treatment include a preliminary period of voice rest. This may be sufficient to resolve the problem or it may need to be used in conjunction with specific voice exercises and techniques to restore full control. Where abuse or misuse is implicated it will eventually be necessary to make long-term changes in voice use and production.

Voice rest does effectively improve a wide range of voice problems where trauma to the vocal cords needs to be reduced. However, in order to produce good results it must be carried out properly by the client, which means adequate preparation by the doctor or communication therapist, with frequent support sessions during the period of rest. It is not sufficient to mention to the client in passing that he needs to stop using his voice. He is being asked to make a drastic change in a very basic behaviour and such long-standing habits cannot be broken overnight or casually.

The very people who need to be on voice rest are often 'talkers' and find even temporary rest very difficult even though motivation may be high. If you are in any doubt about this, try ordering yourself to stop taking for an hour after you have read this. There will probably be all sorts of extremely good reasons why you should put it off for a few hours or until next week, and even why you should not do it at all.

Most dysphonias are treated initially by antibiotics, but these aren't always necessary. Drugs will have no effect on a dysphonia causes by vocal abuse. Shouting, long periods of 'lecturing style' talking, excessive throat clearing, raising the voice above background noise and habitually speaking louder than the situation demands are common culprits and the symptom can only be resolved by easing the strain on the cords and by a change in behaviour. Voice rest acts rather in the manner of a crash diet in that it alleviates the immediate problem, but, for the solution to be long lasting, vocal habits have to be changed.

Vocal nodules

Persistant misuse and abuse lead eventually to the formation of vocal nodules in both children and adults. These are benign lesions of the vocal cords found bilaterally at the junction of the anterior third and posterior two-thirds of the cords (Fig. 6.4). Once established they prevent adequate closure and the voice becomes hoarse and breathy with lower pitch.

It is not usually necessary to remove the nodules surgically unless they are large. Initially further trauma must be prevented by a period of voice rest and eliminating any bad vocal habits. The nodules then decrease in size and disappear with no permanent damage to the cords or deterioration in voice quality. They can be removed surgically although the client will still need retraining in the use of their voice both to minimize the effect of scarring and to prevent recurrence. Repeated surgical procedures of this type will result in a build-up of scar tissue with a consequent reduction in voice quality, stamina and flexibility and therefore it

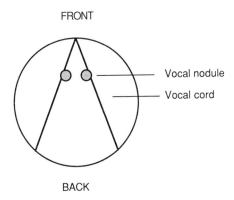

Fig. 6.4 Vocal nodules typically form at the junction of the anterior third and posterior two-thirds of the cords.

is important to make permanent changes in the way the voice is used. Clients treated surgically without voice therapy are more likely to suffer recurrence and a reduction in voice quality than those who do receive voice therapy (Lancer *et al.*, 1988)

PSYCHOGENIC VOICE DISORDERS

Disorders of voice that have a psychological aetiology are very common but are frequently misdiagnosed and confused with organic problems. This is hardly surprising as onset often occurs after some small physical incident such as a cold, breathing in fumes or minor neck surgery, and these occurrences tend to focus the symptom. Psychogenic voice disorders are more common in women than men and rarely present in children under 10 years old.

The larynx is anatomically normal on examination. There may be a history of voice loss but the voice will otherwise have been normal and unless the dysphonia is of long standing, normal voice can still be obtained on coughing or laughing. There may be a current or recent history of emotional distress. The voice is breathy or aphonic but is not usually laboured and does not deteriorate during periods of use. Abnormal pitch levels can be the sole manifestation with phonation remaining relatively undisturbed.

A client with a psychogenic dysphonia/aphonia is someone who is sufficiently stressed for there to be an effect on healthy laryngeal musculature. Although it is not always easy to pinpoint the emotional trigger for the symptoms, classically the choice of conversion symptom is symbolically relevant to the underlying conflict. So someone with a dysphonia might be expected to have some emotional difficulty in expressing what they want or need to say. Frequently, deep seated anger or repressed grief is the cause of the problem and the person may need help in identifying and dealing with these feelings.

It must be stressed that such a person is not consciously simulating the symptom or malingering. His symptoms are real and if he says he is experiencing discomfort or pain then those sensations are there. At some subconscious level he has decided it is easier to express concern over a physical problem than an emotional one.

Having a poor voice may carry some advantages. A child may

be happy to miss school or certain activities, or an adult may enjoy the sympathy and concern of those around them. Both will declare they wish to recover a good voice, but particularly in adults there can typically be a *belle indifférence* to the distress and inconvenience of being voiceless.

I recently came across an old video clip of a colleague interviewing a chatty lady who had a severe psychogenic aphonia. This lady spoke in an effortless whisper and when she was asked how long she had been without a voice replied, 'about fourteen years', smiling all the time as nonchalantly as if she were discussing the weather! It was significant that in all that time she hadn't pressed for any treatment.

If any dysphonia does not respond quickly to medication and there is no obvious vocal abuse or misuse on questioning, then it is likely to be psychogenic or functional. Gross cord movements and structure can be checked in an ENT clinic by laryngoscopy (using a mirror to examine the larynx) or ideally by flexible fibre-optic rhinolaryngoscopy (FFRL). Here a fibreoptic tube is fed through the nose and suspended above the larynx where the moving cords can be observed during phonation. Once the larynx has been shown to be free of any disease the client can be referred for therapy.

Most people with psychogenic voice problems do not require a psychiatric referral. Their dysphonia can be resolved with appropriate counselling and/or symptomatic treatment. The condition responds well and most patients can expect to achieve normal voice within 3–12 weeks. With such clients it is not helpful persistently to treat the voice problem with antibiotics or voice rest. Neither of these will alleviate the condition unless they have some placebo effect. The client has already unconsciously substituted a physical symptom as being more acceptable than identifying and acknowledging the relevant psychological factors and therefore a physical approach to management simply reinforces their own conviction that there is an organic aetiology. This makes it harder to investigate the real causes. Some dysphonics may themselves suspect their voice loss is psychogenic but others will find it hard to accept, insisting they have no anxieties and are not under any stress. The dysphonia may be the result of a build-up of minor stresses or current events may simply be acting as triggers for unresolved conflicts that go back a long way and therefore are not easily identified. On the other hand the symptom may be obviously related to some significant life change which has

103

stretched the person's normal coping strategies. Bringing these unspoken anxieties into the open in the presence of an accepting therapist will begin the resolution of the symptom.

Puberphonia

This psychogenic voice disorder refers to the failure to change to a lower pitched voice in adolescence and consequently the voice stays inappropriately high for the accompanying physique. It occurs in males where normal pitch changes at this time should result in the voice dropping anything up to a full octave.

Puberphonia occurs despite otherwise normal sexual maturation. The structure of the vocal cords is normal and the larynx undergoes the usual physical changes at this time. The angle of the thyroid cartilage becomes more acute, the cords are lengthened and the larynx comes to rest lower in the neck. In puberphonia the larynx is physically capable of producing a deeper voice and automatic laryngeal responses such as coughing and laughing are usually performed at a deeper pitch than that used for speaking.

In an otherwise normal male, puberphonia can indicate a fear of the adult world and a reluctance to take on normal responsibilities such as coping with a job, having girlfriends and dealing with changing relationships and roles within the family. Sometimes the family, and particularly the mother, are protective in a way that does not encourage emotional maturity.

Young men who are puberphonic should be referred for help early and not left for a year or two to see what happens. The longer the symptom and the conditions surrounding it persist, the harder it is to treat. Otherwise it responds well to therapy that identifies and deals with the precipitating fears and at the same time demonstrates the presence and desirability of a normal voice. Puberphonia may sometimes be resolved in just a few sessions, unless the person is very immature or has accompanying psychiatric problems.

ORGANIC OR PSYCHOGENIC?: A DIFFERENTIAL DIAGNOSIS

Table 6.1 provides some pointers towards a differential diagnosis between an organic and a psychogenic dysphonia.

Table 6.1 Differential diagnosis between organic and psychogenic dysphonria

Organic	Psychogenic
Voice deteriorates through the day or over episodes of talking.	Voice may fluctuate but no steady predictable pattern. Often worse in morning. May be a noticeable change while relating some key distressing incident. Voice deteriorates during periods of tension. Commonly, '. . . much better while I was on holiday'.
Voice fluctuates over half an hour or several hours. Any change is gradual. Voice 'tails off'	Changes in voice quality are abrupt. Voice may 'go' in the middle of a sentence. Temporary recovery may be equally abrupt.
Sore throat and/or aching neck by the end of the day or after talking.	No discomfort of note. May be some neck tension by the end of the day.
May be habitual throat clearing.	Client may describe an accompanying lump in the throat, globus hystericus.
Some symptom relief from antibiotics, saline washes, lozenges, etc.	Does not respond to medication except in some cases as a placebo. Tranquillizers, depressants, etc. are not really necessary. The voice symptoms can usually be resolved by communication therapy.
Poor voice on coughing or laughing.	Good strong voice on coughing or laughing.
The client may respond positively to queries about current stresses because the basic organic problem may have a psychogenic overlay, or the pathology may be secondary to some precipitating stress.	Usually does respond positively to queries about current stress sources. However, many people block this and insist they have no such problems but the symptom may be related to previous stress episodes and not consciously identified by the client.
Voice quality is usually strained and hoarse.	Voice is very breathy or the person is aphonic. An easy whisper with no obvious forcing is a sign of a psychogenic disorder. Can be pitch disturbances.

THE VOICE OF THE TRANSSEXUAL

Although transsexuals cannot strictly be considered to have a voice disorder, those who are wishing to change from male to female usually need help to achieve a voice that is appropriate for their appearance. Transsexuals are people who believe that their mind is trapped in the wrong sex body (Wolff, 1977). The aetiology of the condition is not clear but most transsexuals have been aware of their convictions regarding their sex from an early age.

Transsexuals can obviously be of either sex but the hormone therapy administered when the change is from female to male has the effect of thickening the vocal cords and producing a corresponding drop in pitch. When the change is the other way round, things are not so straightforward. The hormone therapy has no direct effect on voice quality and the client has to work hard to use a more appropriate voice.

A lot of this process will centre around the overall pitch of the voice, but pitch is not the only distinguishing feature between male and female speech. Other sex markers such as volume, intonation patterns, vocabulary, use of polite speech forms and differences in assertiveness styles have been suggested as contributing to our perception of whether a person sounds male or female (Coates, 1986). Changing a male voice so that it sounds appropriate for a female body will focus on pitch, volume, voice quality and articulation. The fundamental frequency range for men is in the region of 60–260 Hz and 128–520 for women (Oates and Dacakis, 1983) and thus there is an overlapping frequency band of approximately 128–260 Hz which can represent a normal male *or* female voice (Fig. 6.5). We know from common sense that some women have deep voices and some men have higher, lighter sounding voices. We occasionally misjudge sex on the phone when we have no visual clues to guide us.

The overall pitch of a person's voice is limited by the anatomy and physiology of their vocal tract. Trying consistently to use a higher pitch than a particular vocal tract was designed for will eventually result in voice problems and in any case will sound forced and unnatural, so a balance has to be struck between what is desirable and what is practical and possible. One of the first problems to be overcome is that of the stereotyped ideas held by many transsexuals about how women actually sound., Many have already experimented with their voice before they present in clinic

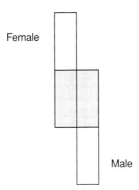

Fig. 6.5 Male and female pitch ranges overlap. The range in the middle is 'normal' for both.

and all too often the result is a pantomine dame falsetto that detracts from, rather than adds to the desired impression.

Voice work aims to shift the pitch to somewhere within the middle neutral range, where the pitch might be classified as being suitable for a man or a woman in order that appearance and behaviour may then hopefully influence the listener towards the desired conclusion.

Within the overall pitch range there are syllable to syllable changes in frequency that make up our intonation patterns. What tends to happen after therapy is that the overall speaking pitch range does not alter greatly, but the higher end of the range is used more frequently, thus giving the impression of a higher pitched voice. The computer histograms in Fig. 6.6. show the frequency distribution during a short spoken passage. The first

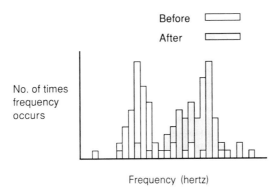

Fig. 6.6 The frequency distribution in the voice of the transsexual client during a spoken passage before and after voice work.

reading was taken prior to therapy, the second after about four months' voice work. It can clearly be seen that the higher frequencies are being used more often in the later trace although the overall range has not altered.

The person wanting to change their voice in this way must be psychologically stable if they are to succeed. It is sometimes assumed that altering a man's voice to sound like a woman's is simply a question of diligently carrying out voice exercises. However the sound of our voice is a key part of our identity in the same way as our appearance. We can be recognized by the unique quality of our voice. Transsexuals have to be willing to alter many aspects of themselves and those who have not reached this stage are unlikely to achieve much in voice therapy. Attempting to force vocal change prematurely will lead the client to reject therapy.

In the UK, achieving an acceptable voice is important not only for social acceptance but because one of the criteria for surgery (in which the male sex organs are removed or modified in order to create an artificial vagina) is that the person lives and supports themself financially as a woman for at least a year. The extent to which they are able to do this successfully depends on their ability to look, act and sound like a woman. So a good acceptable voice is one of the keys that unlocks the door to surgery and while for some transsexuals surgery is not an inevitable end point, for many it is a goal towards which they strive.

SPASTIC DYSPHONIA

This label is usually given to abnormal spasm of the vocal cords on phonation. The spasm is involuntary and intermittent and makes the voice sound strangled, harsh and hard to produce, often with some tremor. Onset is gradual, usually in middle age. In the early stages there may be asymptomatic periods but symptoms are present continuously several months after the initial onset.

Until the 1960s spastic dysphonia was considered to be a particularly intractable form of psychogenic disorder but since then there has been considerable evidence to suggest that some spastic dysphonias may be a focal dystonia involving the laryngeal muscles. Aaronson (1985) describes three types of spastic dysphonia, an adductor type where the cord spasm tends towards the midline (this can have a psychogenic or neurological aetiology), an abductor type with hyperabduction of the cords and a mixed adductor-abductor type. The condition has been notoriously difficult to treat and while the early studies on surgical section of the recurrent laryngeal nerve showed considerable success, later work has questioned its long-term effectiveness. A chemical nerve block is usually employed as a primary procedure to determine whether an particular client might benefit from sectioning but this can be difficult to perform reliably. The first line treatment usually involves a period of voice therapy and the effectiveness of both conservative and surgical treatment varies considerably from client to client.

7

Communication breakdown associated with specific disorders

COMMUNICATION DISORDERS AFTER STROKE

A stroke or cerebrovascular accident (CVA) which involves the speech and language areas of the left hemisphere will cause dysphasia, dyspraxia or dysarthria or a combination of all three. Finding out how much of each is contributing to the communication breakdown is a complicated process, but a differential diagnosis can be made by careful formal testing. When more than one of the above is present, each will complicate the rehabilitation of the other. It has to be stressed again that when someone is dysphasic after a stroke, the dysphasia will have both a receptive and an expressive component, even though the former may not be immediately obvious in general conversation. Conversations are not always demanding. It is possible to manage with the odd 'yes', 'no', a few head nods and some smiles. Testing inevitably demonstrates the presence of a comprehension problem at some level.

In the case of stroke the onset of dysphasia is usually sudden and the client will be bewildered by what has happened to him. It will take a while for him to understand the nature of his disorder as, like most people, he will have had little or no prior contact with it. Many dysphasic stroke victims fear they have gone mad when they regain consciousness and find they are unable to structure their thoughts as before and need extensive reassurance that this is not the case. Most improvement will occur in the weeks and months following the incident, after which the rate of improvement will slow down but there can be significant language improvement for up to a year. After this, although formal language ability is unlikely to change greatly, the way people function in their daily lives can still improve as they adapt to their disabilities, learn to make use of strategies that make full use of their remaining abilities, draw on the full range of their remaining communication skills and gain confidence.

Various factors have been implicated in influencing the recovery process. People with jargon dysphasia tend to do less well than those with non-fluent dysphasia. The more extensive the initial lesion, the more severe the symptoms and the longer the road to recovery. This will be complicated by any concurrent memory, visual or hearing problems. The younger the person when the stroke occurs, the better their prognosis. When very young people, say in their twenties, have a stroke, then improvement occurs over a shorter time period and in addition reaches an end-point nearer to the pre-morbid language level than when the stroke happens in later life. Those with good home support and who live in a stimulating environment where there is an opportunity to retain some responsibility, however small, and where there is something worth talking about, are also more likely to do well. Those clients who display a strong drive towards independence post-trauma will fare better. Occasionally this can be counter-productive as a single-minded determination to recover speech can block the employment of other forms of communication that would otherwise be useful. Those who are able to grieve for their language losses in such a way that they are able to accept their new circumstances (Chapter 9) are more likely to make the most of their residual communication abilities.

A series of small strokes, transient ischaemic attacks (TIAs), can produce what appears to be a gradual diminishing of communicative performance over an extended period of time. The exact effect of each lesion will depend on its site.

COMMUNICATION DISORDERS AFTER CLOSED HEAD INJURY

A closed head injury is one where the injury is a blunt blow to the head associated with acceleration and deceleration forces. Primary damage comes from lacerations and contusions, diffuse and multifocal shearing lesions, tearing of neural tissue and the penetration of tissue by bone fragments. These injuries give rise to some diversity of symptoms. Secondary damage is caused by oedema and raised intracranial pressure, hypoxic ischaemia and haematomas occurring after the original trauma. As the medical

111

and nursing care of head-injured people continues to improve, a population is created of survivors who have some degree of brain damage. As young adults are a high-risk category for head injury, the rehabilitation needs of this population are extensive and long term (Ylvisaker and Szekeres, 1986)

The brain damage sustained may give rise to dysphasia, dyspraxia and dysarthria. As brain injury is more diffuse in head injury than, say, after a CVA, these deficits are compounded by other factors such as memory, perceptual and behavioural problems. Even when there is only a minimal disturbance of formal language or speech, there can be a marked effect on higher communicative processes and the interactional elements of communication may be disturbed. Such people would simply be perceived as having odd behaviour in terms of their non-verbal communication, turn taking, topic handling and other conversational skills. Thus although the formal language ability may remain quite high, the style of communicating is bizarre and any interaction with that person is difficult, as shown in this conversation between a therapist and Roger, who was dysphasic after a head injury sustained when he came off his bike a month previously.

Therapist:	I just want you to tell me a bit about yourself.
Roger:	About myself.
Therapist:	Yeah. Anything you can think of.
Roger:	What do you mean though?
Therapist:	Well, tell me where you live.
Roger:	Castle Road.
Therapist:	Right, where's that?
Roger:	Live at Castle Road.
Therapist:	Yeah?
Roger:	Where's it at now? Er . . . Loxley.
Therapist:	Loxley. Well done.
Roger:	Live at Loxley, yeah.
Therapist:	Yeah.
Roger:	Do you know where Loxley is?
Therapist:	I do, yeah.
Roger:	It's a bit further down than that.
Therapist:	Right.
Roger:	Well, Loxley is a school you see. It's just a bit further down that you see, though it's at Loxley.
Therapist:	Right.
Roger:	Know what I mean?

Therapist:	I do.
Roger:	It's . . . er . . . called Loxley you see.
Therapist:	And who lives in that house?
Roger:	Mum and dad.
Therapist:	Yeah?
Roger:	Who's that now, oh . . .
Therapist:	Have you any brothers or sisters?
Roger:	Sharon.
Therapist:	Yeah.
Roger:	She's . . . er . . . nineteen.
Therapist:	Right.
Roger:	I think she's nine . . . I think she's nineteen.
Therapist:	And how old are you Roger?
Roger:	Seventeen.
Therapist:	Yeah?
Roger:	I think so.
Therapist:	OK.
Roger:	Either seventeen or eighteen. I can't really remember.
Therapist:	OK, it's not that important. And what do you do with your time? Do you work?
Roger:	I do a bit. Yeah. Like at Loxley.
Therapist:	Doing what?
Roger:	That's it . . . Loxley you see. It's like in town, know what mean, do you know what I mean?
Therapist:	No. I'm just getting a bit confused. Do you work in town or in Loxley?
Roger:	Well, it's like . . . you know where Loxley is?
Therapist:	I do.
Roger:	It's there.
Therapist:	Is that where you work?
Roger:	It is. Yeah.
Therapist:	And what sort of work is it?
Roger:	It's just a school you see, as in . . . like . . . it's got a lot of schools. Do you see what I mean? It's called Loxley. It's just like a lot of schools you see.
Therapist:	Do you work at the school?
Roger:	Yeah, it's just called a lot of schools you see.
Therapist:	What do you do there?
Roger:	I just work there you see. I just work a lot of schools you know. What I mean . . . I just work a lot of things, you see.

Therapist: What do you like doing when you're not working?
Roger: When I'm not working, well I work at Lo . . . um . . . school. Not school, sorry. What were they called? I just like to work at Loxley, you know, like on a bike.

Hardly an easy conversation despite the fact that Roger's sentences are usually gramatically correct and he has access to a fair amount of vocabulary, although he does demonstrate some word finding problems. He uses a lot of redundant language and social phrases such as 'you see' that fill some gaps but do not give us any useful information. In fact because they are used in excess they become intrusive and irritating. The exchange provides a good example of perseveration, a behaviour which commonly occurs in dysphasia. Roger gets hooked into a particular word, in this case Loxley, the suburb of Sheffield where he lives, and this word is repeated inappropriately. It is hard to switch off the effect once it has started especially as very often the speaker is not aware of what they are doing. The best way is usually to switch topics completely. If perseveration persists it indicates that the person is tired and needs a break from speaking. Words, phrases and ideas can all be perseverated.

Roger may well be the sort of person who would perform reasonably well on a formal language test and lead us to expect easier and more productive conversations with him than he is able to deliver. How can the formal linguistic abilities of any individual as demonstrated on a test remain relatively intact while the day-to-day performance is so grossly impaired? It has been suggested that the conditions under which formal testing is carried out may in themselves compensate for a client's deficits (Baxter *et al.*, 1985). A quiet and tidy testing area may compensate for attention and concentration problems; short testing sessions may compensate for fatigue and perseveration; tests that do not involve learning avoid difficulties of learning and memory; an unambiguous explanation of tasks compensates for task orientation problems and problem solving; the interactive style of the tester compensates for motivation difficulties and tasks that present less information than real life contexts do not necessarily reveal any general inefficiency in information processing. These higher skills are likely to be the very areas of deficit for head-injured people. Such deficits are more likely to become apparent over a period of observation of the client in a range of environments and situations, so although formal testing is a valuable part of assessment, it has to be carried out in conjunction with observation of communicative and other behaviours over a period of time.

In this transcript, George who had a head injury one year before the tape was made, tries to summarize a story he has just heard.

Well, it's about a man who seems a bit unsure about himself with the betting, picking winners. He's with . . . er . . . about . . . er . . . tax . . . er not tax. Tax on his place. Met an old girl who'd got some money. This old girl had got some money. Got called away from it. He was able to pick some up and put some in his pocket. I assume that he left the place. It doesn't say in the story whether he'd left the place or, what I think it said . . . he went Harry's place but whether it was the same place or a different one I don't know. Assuming it was a different one he seemed as though he was paid for himself for his drinks, his food and whatever. The man he was with seemed to owe him some money but with winning and losing he was no good to take luck for this man to start losing. Plus the fact the money he pinched off Mrs Smith he had pinched off her, so and it was new style money, so keeping that in mind be wary of this sort of man because of his betting, he's likely to be cut out of . . . so you be careful. I understand betting laws and I understand he could lose some. He take some and you win some. You got to work out on that day what you can stand. Whether it's to win or lose. That man did win some. Debatable. The other man had to pay him out. That was debatable whether it was good money or old money because of some painting that had gone off. Assuming that it was good money the old man would pay him money of his own but that was debatable whether it was good or bad. So if it's his own let him get on with it 'cos he knows what he's going to do to it. If that man's son come to take you and the other man outside, that's roughly where the story ended. So they say goodbye. That's it. But the story is basically about a man, his gambling and tax on such places as where you live and where you work.

Most of George's sentences are grammatically correct and he has access to a reasonably adequate vocabulary and yet we find his account extremely hard to follow. There is little organization of the content of his story and ideas are not expressed in a logical sequence. It is almost as if his language is presented externally in an unedited form just as it occurs to him in his head. Much of the language is redundant and he repeats things he's already said. He actually tells us as much in his final sentence as in the whole of the preceding account.

In order for you to make an estimate of George's effectiveness as a communicator, here is a summary of the story he heard:

> Len owes money from gambling activities to a dealer, Harry the Horse. He cannot pay and impersonates a government rates officer in order to raise some quick cash. The occupant of the first house he visits will not admit him without an ID card. At the second house, Mrs Smith invites him in and talks incessantly of her late husband. She offers Len a cup of tea and while she is making it he goes upstairs, finds drawers full of ten pound notes and helps himself to as many as he can carry. He later uses this stolen money to pay off Harry the Horse and places a new round of bets, most of which come up as winners. He prepares to celebrate with a night on the town and meets Harry again. Harry tells Len that the money he used to pay his debts was counterfeit. Meanwhile Mrs Smith is thinking that she needs to go shopping in the morning and remembering how her late husband always told her never to spend more than ten pounds at a time of the money he left her.

As a general rule of thumb it is often said that people who have had CVAs communicate better than they talk, whereas those who have had head injuries talk better than they communicate.

COMMUNICATION DISORDERS IN PARKINSON'S DISEASE

There is general agreement that the incidence of Parkinson's disease increases almost exponentially with age. The cause of the disease appears to be the loss and degeneration of neurones in the dopaminergic systems of the brain, together with a decline in the production of dopamine in the basal ganglia. The principal signs of the disease are tremor, rigidity of muscles, slowness and paucity of movement, poor balance control, as well as difficulty with the initiation and termination of movement. Increased salivation plus difficulty in swallowing leads to drooling.

The combined effect of these deficits is bound to have a significant effect on speech and Selby (1968) found some aspect of speech production was disordered in all the cases he studied, although it was interesting that half of these reported their speech was normal. More recent studies support the idea that speech problems occur in one-half of all cases of Parkinsonism.

Dysarthria is usually considered to be the dominant speech symptom but this is really a simplification of a complex picture. A more comprehensive description of the features of the hypo-kinetic type of dysarthria typically associated with Parkinsonism is given by Darley *et al.* (1969):

1. Monotony of pitch, reduced stress and a monotony of volume;
2. An imprecision of articulation, resulting in a 'blur' of speech;
3. Speech is often arrested, resulting in inappropriate silences and sometimes repetitions of phonemes and syllables;
4. Speech is produced in short rushes. The rate is often variable;
5. Vocal quality is often breathy.

Although the disease is thought of as a disease of movement, there is some evidence of receptive involvement, particularly of spatial and visual perception. This has led to work on the appreci-ation of stress and intonation patterns by Parkinson patients both in their own speech and in the speech of others. The typical facial rigidity which gives rise to a mask-like facial expression also impairs non-verbal communication (Scott *et al.*, 1985). In addition the normal effects of ageing on communication must be taken in to consideration when estimating the impact of Parkinson's disease on any individual's speech.

Management

Drugs usually play the most important part in the management of the symptoms of Parkinsonism, although before the use of levadopa speech did not seem to be much improved by either anticholinergic drugs or surgery. Even with levadopa, speech seems to be less dramatically affected than other physical signs and while there can be some change for the better in articulation, voice quality and intonation, the rapid rate of speech remains unaltered and even by itself may make speech unintelligible.

Unfortunately some drugs administered to Parkinson patients can have an adverse effect on speech. Too high doses of levodopa

117

can cause akinesia and dysphonia, resulting in unintelligible speech; benzodiazepines such as diazepam or nitrazepam can cause increased slurring of speech in high doses while their effect on higher functions can produce an increased use of inaudible or unintelligible remarks. Tricyclic antidepressants may give rise to speech blocks with long pauses being inserted into sentences. The phenothiazines may cause orofacial writhing movements as a side effect, while lithium can cause dysarthria. Phenytoin can cause a cerebellar dysarthria as a side effect of anticonvulsant therapy.

Communication therapy with Parkinson patients aims to maximize the person's residual speech abilities. Historically therapeutic approaches have been geared towards restoring muscle activity through exercise, facilitating sensory responses in order to stimulate a motor reaction, or exercises to achieve increased precision in articulation. Conflicting opinions about the effectiveness of therapy for specific speech features, together with the degenerative nature of the disease, resulted in therapists holding different convictions as to the efficacy of intervention and hence a patchy provision for clients. Studies using more recent methods of therapeutic intervention suggest that some clients can benefit considerably from structured help. Scott *et al.* (1985) recommend that an ideal therapy regimen should be both short term (a minimum of two weeks) and intensive. It should concentrate on respiration, swallowing, facial expression and intelligibility, as well as the client's understanding of intonation, stress and loudness patterns. There is an increasing tendency to do such work in groups, and the results obtained from vacation groups where therapy is carried out in relaxed and congenial surroundings are particularly encouraging, with clients gaining in confidence, motivation, awareness and understanding of their communication problem. Augmenting the person's communication with communication aids may be appropriate and necessary for some.

COMMUNICATION DISORDERS IN MOTOR NEURONE DISEASE

Motor neurone disease (MND) refers to a group of disorders which affect motor neurones in the brain and spinal cord. Motor neurones control muscles and hence movement and so MND causes a wasting and weakness of the muscles involved. It is a progressive disease and usually affects people over the age of forty. If the nerves that control muscles used in speech are affected it will produce a dysarthria. The exact symptoms will depend on whether it is the upper or lower motor neurones that are involved. If it is the upper motor neurones the dysarthria will comprise a spastic weakness of the muscles and imprecise, laboured articulation. There may well be difficulty in coordinating breathing for speech and some degree of dysphonia (spastic dysarthria). Lower motor neurone deficits give rise to wasting and flaccidity of the oral muscles, particularly the tongue and lips (flaccid dysarthria). Again articulation is imprecise, there is some dysphonia and a nasal voice quality due to insufficiency of the soft palate. In both types impairment of the vocal cords prohibits good intonation patterns and speech is monotonous. Both spastic and flaccid dysarthrias may present together. It is sometimes the case that a chronic dysphonia is the very first manifestation of the disease.

As with any dysarthria the client has to learn consciously to control his speech to maintain intelligibility for as long as possible. At later stages of the disease the dysarthria becomes progressively more severe and the client finds himself unable to produce recognizable sounds. A communication aid will help him to retain some communication with others.

THE LANGUAGE OF DEMENTIA

The term dementia covers several conditions that are marked by characteristic memory and intellectual changes. Alzheimer's disease is the most common of the irreversible dementias with multi-infarct dementia (MID) being the second most common. In MID there are numerous transient ischaemic attacks or small strokes, each one adding slightly to the damage caused by the previous ones. This results in a step-like progression of the disease in contrast to the gradual deterioration that is encountered in Alzheimer's disease. The main symptoms are intellectual deterioration and memory impairment but there may also be emotional lability and dyspraxia. Paranoia, hallucinations, decreased attention span, wandering, incontinence and communication breakdown can all be present.

It is possible to see a general pattern in the communication breakdown. Vocabulary is sometimes reduced in the early stages manifesting as a slight word-finding difficulty. As this reduction continues, the use of automatic and social speech predominates until eventually there is marked word finding difficulty,

119

impairment of spoken and written comprehension and an increasing use of jargon. Expression becomes vague and rambling for as the disease progresses the person finds it increasingly difficult to stay with a specific topic. Perseveration, or the inappropriate repetition of words and phrases is common. In the later stages the inability to stick to a relevant sequence of ideas means that the actual content of speech becomes bizarre and distorted with a great deal of repetition.

In the initial stages, some people retain a degree of insight into their failing performance and attempt to cover up their inadequacies by confabulation and indignation and they become anxious about speaking. The person gradually becomes less aware of their conversational partner and the rules of normal conversation are broken. Some people withdraw from communicating, others lapse into jargon.

Making a differential diagnosis between dementia and dysphasia can be difficult, particularly so in the early stages of the disease, because the pattern of language disorganization can be very variable and in addition the two conditions can occur side by side. The term 'the language of dementia' is used to differentiate between the pattern of breakdown found in dysphasia and that found in dementia. There are differences between the two especially when looking at moderate to severe manifestations. In addition the case history and behavioural observations will help to point towards a diagnosis.

The management of the communication problems in the dementing person has to rely on adapting the carer's communication skills to maximize the amount of successful communication that can take place. The carer is asked to modify aspects of their own communication by not changing topics abruptly, restricting the amount of new information given at any one time, slowing the speaking rate, choosing simple vocabulary, using analogy to help comprehension, and being careful with the use of humour and sarcasm.

THE EFFECT OF A HEARING IMPAIRMENT ON COMMUNICATION

There are two main types of deafness. When the ear drum or the small bones of the middle ear are damaged, sound cannot be transmitted to the inner ear. This conductive deafness can often be helped by surgery or by a hearing aid. Conversely the middle ear may be intact but the inner ear or cochlear damaged. The cochlear contains hair cells which stimulate the eighth (auditory) nerve and these hair cells may be damaged or may fail to grow. If enough are left intact, a hearing aid will help. If there are no functioning hair cells or only a few, the person is totally deaf. There are fundamental differences between a total or profound deafness which arises from birth (pre-lingual deafness) and one which comes on later in life after the person has already learned normal speech and language (post-lingual deafness).

The effect of pre-lingual deafness

Many people assume that the main difficulty arising from having a hearing impairment is that of understanding speech and the consequent isolation from the rest of the noise-producing world. However a pre-lingual hearing impairment gives rise to expressive difficulties involving both speech and language.

Language

Where there is a deaf child in the family the parents will naturally have strong desires for the child to speak and understand spoken language. If the child has deaf parents who use sign language from the start, his language development will roughly parallel that of a normal child but many deaf children have parents who do not know for some time that their child is deaf. Prior to diagnosis these children may have many months of exposure to their parents talking that will do little for their language development and at a time that is generally acknowledged to be crucial for language acquisition. This lack of communication may also make it more difficult for an emotional bond to develop and be maintained between the child and its parents (Freeman et al., 1981). Deaf infants begin to make noises at about the same time as hearing children but this then disappears at about six months due to an absence of auditory feedback. There is a tendency for deaf children spontaneously to develop their own gestural systems in the absence of any formal teaching.

Because the pre-lingually deaf person does not learn language primarily through auditory channels like the rest of us, even in adulthood their language may differ from that of a hearing person.

121

The language is limited in its complexity with a restricted and somewhat piecemeal vocabulary. An intelligent pre-lingually deaf girl in her early twenties was familiar with some of the words used to describe some emotions such as 'happiness', 'sadness' and 'embarrassment' but struggled with less common words such as 'jealousy', 'pride' and 'bewilderment'. She then surprised me by easily being able to explain 'ecstasy' as 'extra top happiness'. A very bright deaf boy in his late teens was asked to write some sentences containing the words 'hutch', 'hair', 'reach' and 'relax'. He produced these:

Hutch is the home for rabbits.
My boss always itch his hair when he is listening.
At the moment I cannot reach you for pen.
Scarborough is probably a nice beach to relax for Yorkshire people.

We can certainly understand the meaning of these sentences although the third one may make us pause for thought, yet there is something odd about all of them. The verb tenses are not always correct, the articles a/the are sometimes omitted and occasionally the choice of words is incorrect, as in the use of 'itch' instead of 'scratch' and 'hair' instead of 'head'.

Idiomatic or non-literal speech is often poorly understood by the pre-lingually deaf. We tend to think of idioms as playing a relatively small part in our daily communication and as being fairly obvious figures of speech such as those in the sentence 'That'll put the cat among the pigeons, you mark my words he won't know what hit him'. However, many common words are used extensively in an idiomatic way. A dictionary of English idioms devotes several pages to the use of the verb 'to get', meaning to acquire. For most of us this is a straightforward verb but consider 'to get up, to get on, to get upset, to get by, and to get into'. How do you acquire 'by'? How do you acquire 'into'? We are used to such idiomatic language; it threads unnoticed through our everyday conversations and we understand it both from the context and from our past experience of listening to others. Such illogical language is very difficult for a deaf person to learn. In addition the deaf person has difficulty understanding the speech of others despite the use of lip reading. We all lip read to some extent. Following a conversation when you can't see the speaker's mouth takes a more concentration over a period of time. Lip reading itself is dependent on a good grasp of language.

Speech

The pre-lingually deaf person has no experience of the auditory sensation of sound. Although vocal cords and speech musculature are usually able to function normally, he has no idea how to use them, or what the end product is supposed to be. It is much easier to reproduce a sound by imitating it than it is to use other channels such as diagrams, or written descriptions. So people described as being deaf and dumb are usually not dumb in the true sense of the word. The anatomy and physiology of their vocal tract is capable of producing normal sound but, without hearing, they do not learn to use their larynx and articulators in an organized way. When they do attempt to speak they lack the feedback we all need to tell us from second to second whether we are performing the right manoeuvres accurately. The speech of deaf people varies from being completely intelligible to unintelligible depending on the degree of hearing impairment. Typical distortions include the lack of differentiation between vowels, omission and distortion of consonants, incorrect stress patterns, strained or breathy voice quality, a pitch which is too high or low and volume which is mismatched with the social context of the interaction. Adolescent deaf boys often need help to allow their voice pitch to drop at the appropriate time.

The effect of a post-lingual hearing loss

People can lose their hearing suddenly or gradually and the loss can be partial or total.

Language

When language has already been acquired a hearing loss will not have any significant effect on the use of language. Written language will be sufficient to stimulate and expand on even a basic knowledge of how language works. The person will still be able to think in words and sentences. Comprehension of spoken language will be the main problem.

Speech

Lack of feedback will eventually interfere with speech production and speech intelligibility will deteriorate. This can be minimized with training so that the person uses other ways to monitor speech. Volume is often a problem as most post-lingually deaf people tend to raise their volume to compensate for their own inability to hear themselves. Resonance, pitch range, breath control, speech rate and rhythm can also deteriorate. Consonant clusters are simplified and vowels become distorted. Therapy can control this deterioration to some extent by enabling the person to monitor their own speech. This process is helped by the use of visual feedback and there are many computer systems on the market which translate auditory signals into visual ones. The client can see their speech output on a screen and if necessary match their output with a model, thus building up accurate visual and tactile patterns of movement. Computer devices such as Visispeech are programmed to monitor and display volume, pitch and voicing.

Signing or speech?

The teaching of speech and language to children who are pre-lingually deaf has long been a topic for debate and dispute. Some workers feel that deaf people can only integrate into a hearing world if they are equipped with the same communication skills as everyone else. They argue that deaf people should ideally be able to interact with anyone with whom they come into contact and not only with those people who have learned a sign language. They maintain that all efforts should be made to teach speech as the primary method of communication, and that speech should be the main channel for communicating information to the child.

The opponents to this view are of the opinion that it is vital for the child to acquire an early facility with language in a way which maximizes his linguistic development. Forcing him to do so through an impaired medium can only hinder this and, because we need language to think (internal language), restrict his cognitive and intellectual development. Some of the signing and other non-auditory systems in use today can be classified as languages in their own right. They are much more structured than the non-verbal gestures used by a hearing person and can readily substitute for spoken language and allow for easy fluent communication. Of course this can only take place between two signing individuals. Most educational systems for the deaf employ both approaches but vary as to when each is implemented.

Hearing aids

Amplification aims to make the most of any residual hearing so that meaning can eventually be attached to the noises perceived. All hearing aids have a microphone which converts sound into an electronic signal, an amplifier which strengthens the signal, an earphone or loudspeaker to change the signal back into louder sound, a power source and a volume control. An earmould is made for a particular individual to fit into the external canal of the outer ear. For children these must be re-made to accommodate growth. Hearing aids are not ideal and may have particular limitations in group or noisy conditions because all the sound is amplified and not speech selectively.

Cochlear implants

It was not possible to help people with profound inner ear deafness until the 1970s when cochlear implants were developed. A cochlear implant is a special kind of hearing aid that translates the acoustic speech signal to an electrical one and stimulates the auditory nerve directly to produce the sensation of sound. It is only suitable for people who are profoundly deaf and who cannot be helped by conventional hearing aids.

There are many different types of implant now available but they all share common features. The external part of the implant consists of a microphone, a speech processor, a lead and transmitter. The internal part consists of a receiver and electrode/s. A surgical procedure places the internal parts in position. Single channel implants have one electrode that rests either outside the cochlear on the round window or inside. Multi-channel implants have more than one electrode and are therefore capable of passing more than one signal into the cochlear (multi-channel intracochlear systems). These separate electrodes take signals to different points along the cochlear, corresponding to where different frequencies are picked up in the normal cochlear. Thus electrical impulses relating to the high frequency sounds will be directed to

125

the lower end of the cochlear where high frequency sounds are normally received, while electrodes towards the apex of the cochlear carry more low frequency information. This complex signal gives more speech information than is possible with a single channel device which carries one message and excites all the nerve fibres throughout the cochlear at the same time. Multi-channel implants are more expensive than single channel ones. They promise the best speech discrimination but initial work has used single channel implants to avoid some maintenance difficulties.

Implants are suitable for comparatively few people. Those who may potentially benefit from the procedure are profoundly post-lingually deaf, with no active middle ear infection, and who are in good health with psychological stability and acceptance of their deafness. Early work on implants has tended to select candidates who have experienced normal speech and language development and lost their hearing at some later stage, but some children and young adults with congenital deafness have been implanted in the United States. Some congenitally deafened people do not like their implants and cease to use them. In the adult deafened client, the implant is more likely to re-awaken past memories of speech and help to make the crude signals coming from the implant more meaningful.

Once the implant is in place, an intensive rehabilitation programme is carried out which can last for up to a year. The end result depends on which sort of implant is used but most clients are able to communicate more effectively than before. Nearly all have improved lip reading skills. Some before and after audio recordings sound dramatic. Using implants it has been possible for some deaf people to understand speech without lip reading and even to carry out conversations over the phone, although this can only be achieved with a multi-channel system. Implants can also help the deaf person to detect and discriminate between environmental sounds, to perceive pitch and intonation patterns, volume changes (and hence vowels and consonants), stress patterns, the temporal differences between words, and the number of syllables in a word.

Tinnitus suppressing devices suitable for transmitting signals to the implant have already been developed. Electrical stimulation of the cochlear can suppress tinnitus in a high proportion of cases.

How to improve communication with a deaf person

When someone speaks, clues are gained not only from what is heard but also from what is seen. Simple actions taken can make it easier for a deaf person to understand you. The following strategies seem obvious but it is not easy to remember them whilst caught up in the flow of a conversation.

1. Make sure you face the person.
2. Avoid speaking to them from another room.
3. Do not speak while looking into a newspaper or a book.
4. Do not cover your mouth with a hand, cigarette or pipe.
5. Do not turn your head away while speaking. This is easier said than done and requires some concentration.
6. Gain their attention before you begin to speak. They need to catch the beginning as well as the end of what you are saying.
7. Let them know what the topic of conversation is. They will find it much easier to understand speech if they know the context.
8. Remove sunglasses when speaking so they can receive as many non-verbal clues as possible.
9. Speak clearly and just a little slower than usual. Do not shout. Do not over-exaggerate your mouth movements as this will distort the natural rhythm of speech.
10. Repeat if necessary but after one repetition re-phrase what you are trying to say as some words are harder to lip-read than others.
11. If you are both still struggling, write down key elements in the message. Don't be embarrassed to do this; the deaf person will appreciate your efforts.
12. Remember that just because someone wears a hearing aid does not mean they can hear as well as you can. Hearing aids amplify background noise as well as speech, so everything just sounds noiser.

COMMUNICATION DISORDERS IN CEREBRAL PALSY

This is an enormous topic in its own right but basically whenever the brain damage involves those motor areas that are involved in the production of speech, there will be some degree of communication impairment. The nature and extent of this will depend on the physical deficit and the cumulative effect of limited communicative experience. It is estimated that 60% of the population of cerebral palsied people in the UK have communication problems (Enderby and Philipp, 1986). The damage to the motor cortex itself gives rise to dysarthria and/or dyspraxia and there can be some language delay as a consequence of restricted developmental experience. Occasionally there may be a language disorder directly related to the primary brain damage. There may also be some dysphonia.

Any associated problems such as learning difficulties, hearing loss, visual problems and epilepsy obviously hinder the acquisition and use of sophisticated language and communication.

COMMUNICATION DISORDERS IN MENTAL HANDICAP

Again, a large subject and one which can only be covered briefly here. Mentally handicapped children have difficulty in learning and using all aspects of language which, as we have seen, comprises high order skills and sophisticated symbolic functioning. There will be varying degrees of language delay and attempts to help such children have to take into account their developmental status and prognosis. Any concomitant physical disabilities will complicate the picture. Some children can be helped towards a basic language competence by gesture systems such as Makaton, which can supplement and extend their existing language.

COMMUNICATION PROBLEMS IN MENTAL ILLNESS

Many mental illnesses can be considered to have some element of disturbed communication. Dementia and elective mutism have been covered elsewhere but other significant conditions include schizophrenia and depression.

Features of schizophrenic communication

1. The language is not used mainly for passing information;
2. Abnormal prosody;

3. There may be preoccupation with particular topics and perseveration of ideas in both speaking and writing;
4. Disordered syntax, telescoping of ideas, idiosyncratic word associations;
5. Disorientation of time, place or person which is reflected in the language. The person confabulates;
6. Poor self-monitoring and short-term memory. The person is easily distracted;

The above impairments are usually taken as reflecting the thought disorder and to be a consequence of the disorganized and bizarre thinking strategies, but it is possible that the language disorder may be the primary one and influence the thought processes.

This letter by a schizophrenic person is quoted by Ailuano Arieti in '*Understanding and Helping the Schizophrenic*' (1981).

Dear Dr Arieti

It is because I Am So Passionate That They Brought Me Here. Doctor Webster Asked Me Why I was Brought Here And I Couldn't Answer Without A Certain Hesitation, But Now I Know, I Know Now:
I'm Too Passionate!
Thats Why I Can't Get A Job.
You Had The Wrong Diagnosis.
Take This For Instance.
Look Up The Word Passions In The Encyclopaedia (A Masterpiece Of A Word) And In The Dictionaries. Don't Get Cerebral Meningitis In Your Studies. But You Will Find That There Is A Difference Between The Passions Of Jesus of Bethlehem And The Passions Of Blue Beard. Between The Passion Of Misplaced Symphonies And The Passions Of Suicidal Thoughts. Are You Passionately In Sympathy With Your Great Poet Dante, Doctor Arieti?
And Am I In Passionate Admiration Of The Works Of Moliere, The French Troubadour.
And There Is The Passion Flower.
And The Passion Plays of Oberammergau.

Depression

Language in depression is usually intact but the content can be restricted and unimaginative. The motivation to communicate is reduced. Intonation patterns tend to be less extensive and the voice in general can be described as flat and inexpressive.

8

Fluency disorders

STUTTERING OR DYSFLUENCY?

There is no such thing as completely fluent speech unless you are reading aloud from a book or quoting lines learned in a play. Normal speech is not fluent because it contains many repetitions, hesitations and pauses. Despite this the majority of people would not class themselves as being stutterers. The label is usually given to those who have become aware of their dysfluencies and are discomfited by them. The term 'stammering' is often used in place of 'stuttering'. Jerky and hesitant speech may frequently be heard in young children between two and four years of age. The child does not usually show any awareness of this and is said to be *dysfluent*. Repetitions of whole words and other minor dysfluencies are quite common but they are normal and their presence should not be allowed to precipitate panic in the parents.

The terms dysfluency and non-fluency tend to be used interchangeably to refer to those speech disruptions when the person is not showing awareness of them, or displaying any secondary features. It is generally considered to be the presence of an emotional response and the onset of avoidance which distinguishes stuttering proper from early dysfluency.

Fluency can be thought of as a continuum with the hypothetical concepts of total fluency at one end and total dysfluency at the other. Even for an individual, fluency levels are not stable and depend on such factors as tiredness, anxiety, confidence and listener reaction. Any child or adult speech will show this variation including that of people who stutter.

AETIOLOGY OF STUTTERING

Stuttering is a complex disorder and research findings relating to its nature and aetiology are inconclusive. No two stutterers have exactly the same overt symptoms or the same attitudes towards communication. A summary of the better established theories is presented below. In addition it is worth noting that:

- there can be a familial tendency to stutter;
- there is a significant incidence of expressive language problems among children who are dysfluent;
- some dysfluent people also have difficulty producing the accurate motor sequences and fine coordination necessary for speech;
- parental reactions do not cause dysfluency, although certain behaviours such as criticism or anxiety may perpetuate existing stuttering symptoms.

Organic theories

There is a strong possibility that some stutters have an organic basis but research data is contradictory.

Neurological

The search for neurological abnormalities has proved inconclusive. It is suggested that there is a connection between handedness and stuttering and that people with crossed laterality, and hence incomplete cerebral dominance or bilateral representation of speech, are more likely to stammer. This notion is still popular although there is little documented evidence to suggest that cerebral dominance does have a significant effect on the development of dysfluency. Some adults who suffer brain damage as a result of stroke or head injury develop a stutter which can be either temporary or permanent.

Auditory feedback

This theory suggests stuttering is caused by faulty bone conduction and hence impairment of the auditory monitoring system for connected speech. A normal speaker will become dysfluent while talking if his own speech is played back to him a fraction of a second later than this normally occurs (delayed auditory feedback). The same will happen when he is deprived of normal feedback by an alternative method which consists of masking with white noise (a random jumble of sounds) which is played directly into the speaker's ears.

Conversely, stutterers subjected to the same process become instantly fluent, a phenomenon which gave rise to the Edinburgh Auditory Masker (EAM), a device which feeds white noise through headphones worn by the stutterer. The noise is synchronized with phonation which is picked up by a small throat microphone. Every time the stutterer beings to speak, the white noise begins, feedback is masked and fluency increases. The effect stops when the masker is removed and in practice EAMs seem to have limited functional use. As they are an obviously visible piece of gadgetry many stutterers do not like to use them. They help severe stutterers in specific situations such as speaking on the phone.

Psychological theories

Behavioural disorders

Several approaches suggest that stuttering develops through classical and operant conditioning. The child learns to stutter because the parents or significant others establish high standards for communication which the child cannot realistically be expected to meet. At the same time they react with disapproval and anxiety to the child's normal non-fluencies, producing anxiety and guilt in the child. Delaying and avoidance speech behaviours are then used by the child to escape unfavourable reactions from others. The parent's negative reactions increase and the cycle of events is fixed. It appears that parental anxiety and correction undoubtedly plays a part in the development of stuttering in many young children. Alternatively the stuttering behaviour may become established and reinforced because the child gains attention during episodes of normal non-fluency and in fact may gain more attention when he is non-fluent than when he is fluent.

Personality disorders

There is little evidence to support the idea that personality and fluency problems are linked, but many covert reactions subsequently develop as a consequence of the initial non-fluency. Frustration, approach/avoidance conflicts and poor conversational skills commonly form a large part of the stuttering complex. Many stutterers feel their stutter has hindered the development of their personality, work and social life. Modern treatment of stuttering acknowledges the importance of the covert symptoms of stuttering and works on these through counselling and psychotherapy.

Linguistic theories

The existence of abnormal language patterns in studies of early stutterers gives some evidence for the implication of linguistic factors in the aetiology of some stutters. It is also known that some stuttering children use less complicated language and have a more restricted vocabulary than non-stutterers. This may be because stuttering children talk less than their fluent peers and therefore have less verbal experience. It can be noted that the onset of normal non-fluency often occurs at an age when the child is also developing competent use of his native language.

FACTORS IN THE DEVELOPMENT OF STUTTERING

While research remains inconclusive as to the aetiology of stuttering, it is accepted that some specific factors may be relevant. These can be considered as those factors which either predispose, precipitate, or perpetuate the stutter.

Pre-disposing factors

1. Familial history of stuttering;
2. Familial history of late language development;
3. Incoordination of the rapid oral movements necessary for good articulation.

Precipitating factors

Physical or emotional trauma such as unexpected separations in the child's life or traumatic early school experiences.

Perpetuating factors

1. High parental expectations of speech performance;
2. Stress at home;
3. Negative reactions of the family to non-fluency such as criticism or anger.

FEATURES OF STUTTERING

Every stutterer could write a different recipe for his own stutter even though these will have some common features. Any individual stutter can be described in terms of its component behaviours.

Repetitions

These may be repeated sounds, words or phrases.

- b . . . b . . . book.
- I bo . . . bo . . . bought a book.
- I bought . . . I bought a book.
- I bought a book . . . I bought a book for a present.

Prolongations

A consonant may be extended beyond its normal length.

- I went ffffive times.

Blocks

A consonant is blocked part of the way through its production and either no sound at all or a distorted sound is produced. The stutterer seems to be 'frozen' into the sound.

- I bought a b . . .

Substitutions and avoidance

A different sound or word is chosen instead of the one that is causing the trouble.

- I bought a b . . . something to read.

This may happen without the listener realizing that a swap has been made (substitution). Words that are anticipated as causing problems may be avoided altogether as may whole situations.

'I never ask for two pints, it has to be one or three. I'd have
a different drink if a friend wanted me to buy him a pint.'
Telephones are particular causes of fear and avoidance.
'I don't ever answer the phone if I don't know who's calling.'

Concomitant movements

Verbal and vocal dysfluencies are often accompanied by facial grimaces, foot tapping, eye movements, banging hands on legs, head jerks, etc. These are probably initiators; the stutterer feels they help him to get going again. They eventually become incorporated into the stuttering behavioural pattern and become part of it, even when they have lost their effectiveness as initiators.

Eye-contact

This is frequently misused by stammerers. They either avoid eye-contact and appear shy or even shifty, or go to the other extreme and adopt an intense stare which is equally inappropriate.

Breathing

During stuttering episodes breathing is poorly coordinated with phonation and phrasing. It is associated with extreme and visible tension in the thorax, neck and facial muscles.

COVERT AND OVERT STUTTERING

Most of the above features produce an obvious effect. The stutter is overt and we can hear the resultant distortion of normal speech. With a covert stutter there may be little or no obvious audible dysfluency but there is considerable disruption of the person's communicative behaviour.

Covert stutterers sometimes have difficulty convincing doctors that they do stutter and hence obtaining a referral for help may not be easy. The open referral system in the UK means that some clients can sidestep this difficulty and contact a therapist directly. A classic covert stutterer could not be detected stuttering in a normal conversation, at least no more than any normal speaker. He would avoid telling friends and colleagues that he stuttered and would go to some length not to get himself into situations likely to promote dysfluency, where he might be found out. One 45-year-old covert stutterer described how in 20 years of supervising a busy typing pool, she had managed never to read aloud to any of her senior or junior colleagues.

Nevertheless the covert stutterer is greatly disturbed by his feared dysfluency and it dominates his interactions with other people. He is an avoider *par excellence* and lives with the fear of being discovered. He frequently feels his stutter has had a negative effect on his life as regards choice of career and relationships, and may blame his past misfortunes or failures on the stutter rather than on other limitations or circumstances.

Covert stuttering symptoms can be represented as a floating iceberg with most of the symptoms hidden below the water level, whereas with an overt stutter we need to imagine an iceberg floating well up in the water with the bulk of the symptoms being clearly visible (Fig. 8.1).

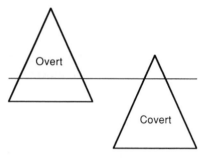

Fig. 8.1 Overt stutterers have obvious symptoms. In covert stuttering many of the symptoms are hidden.

THE REMEDIATION OF STUTTERING

This would usually consist of all or some of the following:

- identification/description of the stutter and awareness building;
- fluency control;
- communication skills training;
- anxiety control;
- counselling/psychotherapy.

Identification of the stutter and awareness building

It is not possible for someone to change a behaviour until they have identified just what that behaviour consists of. A complex and automatic behaviour such as stuttering has to be broken down into its component parts and this can be achieved by the stutterer making and watching video recordings of himself. This process also allows for some desensitization to occur as the stutterer is confronted with aspects of his own dysfluency that he may not have been aware of previously or that he may have tried to ignore. He has to acknowledge and accept his own stuttering behaviour as a starting point for change. This is in direct contrast to the management of young children who are at risk of becoming stutterers. At this stage the more the child gains awareness of his speech, the more likely he will become fearful in speaking situations and so it is important to avoid making the child self-conscious and aware that his speech is in any way different or wrong. At the same time it may also be necessary to work directly on modifying his speech. These two objectives can seem contradictory and management has to be finely balanced.

Fluency control

Achieving an initial temporary improvement in fluency is relatively easy to accomplish using one of a number of techniques which modify the style of speaking. Maintaining such a change in the long term is much more difficult. Techniques commonly used to increase the fluency of both children and adults include the following.

Block modification

This is a complex technique. It attempts to change only those parts of speech that are dysfluent and it is more suitable for people who already have some insight into their problem or the potential to develop it. Block modification is not usually suitable for very severe stutters. It can take longer to master than the other methods but has better long-term prospects. It is a good technique for those prepared to take responsibility for their own speech.

Easy stuttering

Here the stutterer is told to stutter deliberately in order to relieve the tension associated with the usual response of trying to prevent the stutter from occurring. Easy stuttering often removes the secondary characteristics of stuttering such as concomitant movements, facial grimaces and avoidance and, although the core dysfluency remains, nevertheless the speech sounds relaxed and much more normal.

Slowed speech and prolonged speech

These two techniques are very similar though not identical. They both slow the rate of speech and make it smoother. They change the whole speech pattern rather than just the stuttered segments and speech can sound dreary and expressionless. They are popular techniques but slowed speech has superseded prolonged speech as the end result sounds less distorted. Either can produce a dramatic change in fluency, especially if taught intensively.

Maintenance is often a problem and sometimes listener reactions are not positive. Some listeners say they would rather hear the stutter than the slowed speech. It is a good choice for more severe stutters or people with poor insight.

Syllabic speech

This is an old-fashioned method and can be counter-productive. The normal stress and rhythm patterns of speech are suppressed and speech is produced one syllable at a time. 'All-the-syll-a-bles-are-ex-act-ly-the-same-and-the-speech-sounds-mo-no-to-nous-and-stil-ted.' It may aid fluency in some cases but gives rise to negative listener reaction and hence many stutterers do not use it outside a clinic. It can promote head nodding and other undesirable secondary behaviours.

Communication skills training

Many stutterers have poor non-verbal and conversation skills such as eye-contact, turn-taking, listening and giving feedback. They often perceive themselves to be good listeners, a role which they feel has been forced on them as a result of their dysfluency. This is usually not the case as they are too preoccupied with the listener's reaction to them and with their own fear of embarrassment really to be good listeners. They spend time planning and mentally rehearsing their next sentence or negotiating an avoidance rather than participating in the general flow of the conversation.

Both children and adults can be helped to develop better abilities and are given increased confidence by group work on communication and social skills. With children who show early stuttering behaviour, it is important that the family isolates and identifies those factors which are likely to be perpetuating the stutter because the more prolonged the child's experience of non-fluency, the greater the awareness and fear and the greater the likelihood of the dysfluency becoming stabilized. Early identification helps the family to modify their interaction sufficiently to prevent the development of a full-blown stutter.

Counselling

Again this may be employed on its own but more commonly it is combined with a fluency technique. It is necessary because whatever the cause of the core dysfluency, many stutterers appear to resist fluency even when they have mastered a technique that gives them the means to be fluent. The stutterer needs to change his perceptions of himself from 'I am a stutterer' to 'I am a normal speaker'. It frequently adopts a behavioural approach to dealing with the anxieties surrounding the dysfluency and uses desensitization techniques to address specific speaking situations.

Parent counselling is nearly always a vital part of the management of a young stutterer. It is necessary to establish a relationship with one or preferably both parents in which they can express their feelings about the child and his speech. The parents need to understand the normal process of language development and how environmental influences such as competition in speaking, having to talk in threatening situations or talking to an unresponsive listener can affect the child's fluency. Unhelpful family reactions to the dysfluency which might perpetuate the symptoms or decrease fluency even further need to be prevented. It is essential that the family are cooperatively involved; parents who see it as the therapist's responsibility to cure the child are unlikely to see swift results.

Older children can be counselled directly. They can be helped to explore their own negative perceptions of speaking and to reduce the fear and avoidance associated with communicating.

TREATMENT OF SECONDARY STUTTERING FEATURES

Regardless of the type of stutter, secondary behaviours and attitudes build up around the original dysfluency. The following areas would have to be considered in any comprehensive treatment alongside techniques for fluency control.

Anxiety reduction

This is not often used on its own but is usually incorporated into an eclectic approach. It is based on the theory that suggests stuttering is a behaviour aimed at avoiding speaking and the more a stutterer is dysfluent in a particular situation, the more he/she will try to avoid it. Telephones in particular are the cause of much avoidance behaviour. Thus therapy aims to reduce fears of speaking using a behavioural approach in which desensitization strategies, relaxation and role-play techniques are a common feature.

As well as avoiding situations, stutterers avoid specific words and sounds that they know from past experience will cause them problems, substituting safe words and sounds instead. For this reason stutterers who speak a second language appear to be more fluent in their native language because their vocabulary is more extensive and substitutions can be made more smoothly.

People who stutter often ask if hypnosis can help. This depends on the type of stutter. If there is a large anxiety component then hypnosis may help and is worth trying. Most communication therapists now use deep relaxation and hypnotic techniques with stutterers but some stutterers may prefer to work with a hypnotherapist. This approach is often attractive because it appears to require little effort on the client's part and to deliver results relatively quickly. The stutterer needs to be taught auto-hypnotic techniques in order to maintain any benefit. For the majority of stutterers hypnosis is more wisely used as part of an integrated approach involving the elements described above.

Variability

The context in which we interact has an effect on how we perform. All speakers perform better when they are relaxed and in control. This particularly applies to stutterers whose level of fluency varies considerably depending on the situation. Understanding this effect can help to control it. It is important to help the stutterer discover that the anxiety level of normal speakers also varies depending on the situation. Stutterers often have unrealistic ideas about what it is like to be a normal speaker and expect any normal speaker to be able to stand up and address a hall full of people without turning a hair. They also need to be aware that a certain degree of dysfluency is normal and desirable. We are only completely fluent when reading aloud or quoting lines learned by heart, otherwise normal speech contains lots of hesitations, stops, starts and pauses. Listen to normal conversations between people (not scripted conversation on the television) and see how many stuttering features you can spot in their speech. Examine your own speech in the same way. Stutterers are inclined to perceive any such perfectly normal phenomenon as being abnormal when occurring in their own speech and consequently may be expecting more of themselves than they or anyone else could possibly achieve.

The actual fluency levels of a stutterer may even fall within a normal range. While joining in with a group of stutterers during a speaking exercise, I gave a far less fluent performance than any other member of the group. This was not done on purpose. I was simply tired and not giving the job my full attention. I subsequently suggested to the group that they should classify me as a stutterer but they would not accept this. Nor could they accept the alternative logical stance that, on the basis of my speech, they should be re-classified as normal speakers. After some discussion the group decided there was a crucial difference in how I felt about my dysfluencies, in that I was not concerned by them and regarded them as normal, whereas any other member of the group giving the same dysfluent performance would experience a sense of failure and some anxiety.

Attitudes

It is difficult for stutterers to hold their own in the speed and competitiveness of social situations. They are frequently regarded as being less intelligent than their fluent counterparts and may be discriminated against in the job or career market. Regardless of the person's actual suitability for a job, an interview will prove a real hurdle as most stutterers present badly in this situation.

EFFICACY OF REMEDIATION

The timing of intervention can be an important factor as stutterers report long-term fluctuations in their fluency over months or years. When other aspects of life are going well or are stable then fluency is likely to increase. Fluency may decrease during episodes of change or stress. Stutterers often ask for help at these low points. It is relatively easy to improve a person's fluency level especially if the intervention is intensive. Significant changes can be demonstrated in confidence and fluency after a fortnight's full-time group work. Before and after videotapes made on these occasions can look very impressive. However, stabilizing fluency and generalizing it outside a therapeutic setting is much more difficult and many stutterers never successfully negotiate this stage. Maintenance of the new-found fluency is a real problem and many people need formal support over long periods.

As indicated, not all the therapy is geared towards changing fluency. It is sometimes desirable to change the stutterer's attitudes towards his existing level of fluency and towards himself. Otherwise he is unlikely to sustain any improvement made. Such attitude change is a long-term business and should be viewed in terms of months or years. There is no cure for stuttering but the symptoms may be alleviated sufficiently so that it no longer dominates someone's life. Those stutterers who want the therapist to provide a quick cure and all the answers are going to be disappointed and those who enter therapy because their parent, teacher, partner or employer has told them to are unlikely to benefit greatly. On the other hand, those who are willing to confront their disorder, put in the necessary time and effort and take responsibility for its resolution can reap very significant gains.

IMPROVING COMMUNICATION WITH A STUTTERER

1. Generally aim for a relaxed atmosphere.
This will help you as well as the stutterer. It will give him a chance to be as fluent as he is able. Make sure you appear calm as he will usually be aware of your embarrassment.

2. Don't hurry the conversation.
It helps to say things like 'Slow down', 'It's OK, relax', 'Take your time'. Let him finish before you start talking. Avoid interrupting until he has finished.

3. Give feedback.
There may be pauses when neither you nor the stutterer are quite sure what is going to happen next. Use nods and eye-contact to signal that you are still listening. This is particularly important on the telephone; if there is a long block you might need to say something like 'It's OK, I'm still here'.

4. Don't anticipate and supply the ends of sentences.
Even if you feel pretty sure you know what he is going to say you may still be wrong and the stutterer has to start all over again.

Most stutterers report this as the single most infuriating thing normal speakers do to them.

5. Avoid performance tasks.
These are especially daunting for children. Teachers should never force children who stutter to read aloud in class. They are likely to be much more dysfluent when reading aloud because they cannot avoid tricky words and the pressure of an audience sets the scene for humiliating failure.

6. Allow them to have their speaking turn.
In the fast cut and thrust of a conversation it can be hard for a stutterer to have his turn as the actual initiation of a comment is slow. Allow a longer pause for him to take up his turn.

7. De-fuse difficult silences.
This can be done by friendly eye-contact but do not overdo it. If a block or repetition goes on for a long time eye-contact can easily turn into a fixed stare. Go with what feels comfortable. Humour can sometimes work well, in fact the stutterer himself may well help you out by introducing some witty aside. It is acceptable to laugh if given 'permission' in this way. It enables both of you to have some relief.

9

Emotional problems associated with communication disorders

Communication is central to our emotional and social well-being. It is possible to make a distinction between communication problems which are the *result* and those which are the *cause* of emotional distress. Although in practice it is simplistic to separate these two groups we can consider them individually.

COMMUNICATION DISORDERS AS A RESULT OF EMOTIONAL CONFLICT

Voice disorders

Disorders of voice that have a psychological aetiology are common. Unlike other conversion symptoms they usually present in communication therapy clinics following referral from an ENT department, rather than in psychiatric or psychology clinics. Once organic disease has been ruled out, management may focus either on the resolution of the symptoms and/or on their psychological origins. The predominant symptom is usually a breathy effortless dysphonia or even aphonia but there are many variations on this. Sometimes the client has the sensation of having a lump in the throat, globus hystericus, which cannot be dislodged by coughing or swallowing.

A person with a psychogenic voice disorder is someone whose coping mechanisms are sufficiently hard pressed for there to be an undesirable effect on otherwise healthy neuromuscular systems. Classically the choice of conversion symptom is seen as being symbolically relevant for the sufferer and it is sometimes possible to pinpoint a specific trigger for the symptoms. Either way, the person has some emotional difficulty in expressing what he wants or needs to say. Frequently deep-seated anger or grief is the cause of the problem and the person needs help in identifying and expressing these feelings.

It must be stressed that the client is not consciously 'putting on' the symptom, it is real and, for him, uncontrollable. If he says he experiences pain then that sensation is there, but subconsciously he finds it easier to express his anxiety over a physical problem than its emotional cause.

The stress that produces such an effect can be thought of as either externally or internally generated. Externally generated stress occurs when environmental events push an individual's normal coping strategies beyond their limits. This may happen when a person is confronted with a new and unfamiliar experience or simply because the magnitude and number of stressful events is too great to be accommodated by old and previously successful mechanisms. Thus some clients may develop a dysphonia as a reaction to a bereavement or other loss or as a way of coping with significant life events. Internally generated stress arises from the pressures we put on ourselves as a result of our own expectations, attitudes, beliefs, and our personality. So someone with perfectionist tendencies who cannot conceive of a different more accepting way of being, may have unrealistic expectations of their own performance and push themselves to the point of illness, this being a more acceptable alternative to what they would see as failure. Very often it is the interplay of both internally and externally generated stresses that produces a physical effect as the two following histories illustrate.

Audrey was in her late twenties and had had no voice at all for eight months although nothing was wrong organically on examination. She was separated from her husband who had refused to give her a divorce. She had a new relationship and was setting up house with the new partner who was urging her to hurry things along. Audrey anticipated having to wait anything up to five years to obtain her freedom although it could come at any time during this period. She dared not express her anger towards her husband at his behaviour as she felt it would only result in him delaying the divorce even longer, yet her apparent passivity angered her new partner. Consequently she felt trapped and frustrated by her situation and overwhelmed by feelings that whatever she said or did would be unacceptable to someone. Her voice returned after two months of therapy which dealt with her feelings towards her husband and her frustration at her predicament.

Kate was a woman in her early forties who complained of a sudden and complete voice loss. There was no pain although she had the uncomfortable sensation of a lump in her throat. The ENT consultant noted she was a teacher who had recently returned to work after a period at home to bring up three children. He therefore reasonably assumed the problem was one of vocal abuse and referred her to therapy for voice strengthening exercises.

In the initial interview the teaching load emerged as minimal, less than two days a week, and unlikely to account for the current extent of the dysphonia. Kate presented as an intelligent person with some degree of insight. In a forced whisper she described how she enjoyed her children but was now looking forward to being involved in her career again. The present voice loss was threatening this plan. At one point in the session Kate made some reference to a busy schedule and the long waiting times at hospital clinics. As I had not personally kept her waiting I invited her to expand. She regularly accompanied her third child, who suffered from a bone disease, to a hospital clinic. She resented the time spent waiting to see the doctor and often felt tearful during this time without understanding why, as she was happy with the care the child had received and she spoke highly of the consultant involved. She wished her husband, Michael, would take the child to clinic occasionally, but felt unable to ask him to interrupt his work as he was 'generally so good' about sharing tasks. Kate felt she had to take responsibility for this child as she had talked Michael into agreeing to a third baby and felt that she had no right to ask for extra help. Although they had talked through the issues of guilt and responsibility at the child's birth, it was a long time since these had been discussed. Kate had gradually assumed care of the child and this was now conflicting with her wish to work outside the home.

The relationship appeared to be a strong and supportive one and when I asked Kate if she felt able to tell Michael about the things we had talked through in the session, she agreed to think about it. The following week she returned with a normal voice. They had talked things through and agreed that Michael would take more responsibility for the care of the handicapped child. Six months later her voice was still strong and she was easily coping with the teaching load.

Sometimes emotional stress results in an organic pathology. A person who abuses his voice and causes physical damage to the vocal cords does so because of the way he interacts with his environment. It was important for Ken to be macho, one of the boys, and he had developed a lifestyle accordingly. He had been a drill sergeant in the army, he refereed at football matches and prided himself on his authoritative style and having a voice that 'carried'. He smoked and drank to excess and now in his fifties had developed vocal nodules. He found it hard to accept that his expectations of what a normal voice could cope with were unrealistic and felt instead that his voice was weak and letting him down.

Stuttering

In the previous chapter we looked at the many different and sometimes conflicting theories as to the aetiology of stuttering, which make it impossible categorically to state the cause of this complex disorder. Sheehan's approach–avoidance theory suggests that an emotional conflict related to communicating actually provokes the initial dysfluency. The person is ambivalent about speaking; he wants to talk but is afraid to do so.

Elective mutism

This is a disorder in which 'the child refuses to speak in certain circumstances and speaks normally elsewhere (usually at home)'. It affects between 0.3–0.9 children per 100 000 population and nearly all the literature refers to children of school age.

Children with this disorder often show other signs of emotional maladjustment but it is important to differentiate between children with elective mutism and those who are schizoid. There is no direct correlation with any one factor and the disorder appears to have a mixed aetiology including maturational, genetic, parental personality and learned behaviour factors.

Authors are cautious in their estimates for prognosis. Younger children seem to fare better but there is little evidence to suggest that therapy, whether psychotherapy, behaviour modification or communication therapy is generally effective (Kolvin and Fundudis, 1981).

COMMUNICATION DISORDERS WHICH CAUSE EMOTIONAL DISTRESS

The main group to be considered here is that of acquired communication problems. When a person suffers from an acquired dysphasia, dyspraxia, dysarthria or a permanent dysphonia (e.g. after laryngectomy), their previous communicative ability is lost and the tremendous effort involved in communicating feels a poor alternative to normal speech. It has far-reaching consequences and should be seen as a major traumatic event. The emotional reaction to it is intense and long term. For people with acquired brain damage there may also be a concurrent loss of mobility, physical dependence and social change, and the effect of these combined changes is often underestimated. The emotional distress following communication handicap can be viewed as a reaction to loss.

Loss and grieving

A parallel can be drawn between a bereaved person and one with an acquired speech or language handicap. The loss of communication preludes many other losses as a consequence of restricted speech and language. These losses broadly divide into three groups (Tanner and Gerstenberger, 1988).

1. Loss of loved ones in a psychological separation resulting from the communication impairment, as communication is vital for establishing and maintaining relationships.
2. Loss of self implicit in loss of function. There is an inability to perform as before. The point at which awareness of loss of function occurs marks an important stage in the emotional response to the loss. With head injury and other brain damage it may be a while before the person has the perceptual and cognitive ability to be aware of this.
3. Loss of external objects and their symbolic meanings. Owning a car may symbolize freedom and independence even though the person can no longer drive it. Placements in hospital wards, stroke units and nursing homes all entail many object losses.

Grief is defined by the Shorter Oxford Dictionary (1973) as

'Deep or violent sorrow caused by loss or trouble; keen or bitter regret or remorse'. The grieving process itself has been described as a series of events which follow each other in a pattern. There are several different models of this but most contain the features of denial, frustration, depression and acceptance (Tanner and Gerstenberger, 1988). Alternatively the person may move within a cluster of emotions at the same time and then eventually move through the sequence.

These features can be applied to the grief faced by a person who has lost their communication ability.

Denial

This is usually the first stage and may be related to the site of the lesion in some cases. Alternatively it may hold true that some types of communication disorder are more easily recognized by the sufferer than others so the denial may not necessarily be due to psychological factors. Denial can last for a considerable time and serves as a buffer to psychological pain, while giving time to mobilize less radical defences. Denial may manifest itself as a number of different responses.

'I don't believe it.'
'I haven't got a problem, it's the listener's fault.'
'I have a problem but it's minor and/or temporary.' (partial denial)
'I have a significant problem but it's temporary and God/Medicine will make me whole again.' (passive denial)
'I have a significant problem but I will overcome it by hard work and determination.' (existential denial).

Tanner also makes the observation that denial is hard to deal with as it cuts to the core of the helper or therapist role, eliminating any of the helper's credit for improvement.

Frustration

This occurs at the point where the person realizes he can no longer communicate as well as before. He also becomes aware he has no ability to alter the course of events which led to this situation and hence is confronted with unwanted realities which he cannot change. Anger is the commonest reaction to frustration but where there is a communication handicap it can be difficult to express this anger adequately or appropriately. When there is poor command of words, a slow delivery and no ability to raise the volume of voice, the anger experience is drastically changed.

Bargaining is another reaction to frustration and can be done either with therapists, God or medicine. To some extent bargaining also denies the extent of the disability. Bargaining responses would be:

'If I try hard enough I'll overcome it.'
'If I have more therapy I'll overcome it.'

Unnecessary collusion with such bargaining may interrupt the normal progression of the grief process.

Depression

When the person's defences are no longer able to buffer or delay awareness of his loss, depression occurs and may last for days or months. This is a normal reaction and only becomes pathological when the duration or severity of the response exceeds normal limits. Unfortunately some people do not move beyond this stage.

Acceptance

This is the ultimate goal of normal grieving, where the loss is accepted as neither good nor bad but just the way things are and when the person is able to gain some emotional distance from the loss. Tanner stresses that this is not the same as resignation where the client tolerates the situation because there is nothing they can do about it. Sometimes the fatigue, apathy and withdrawal associated with depression can be neurogenic. Post-stroke depression can last for anything between one to two years post-onset. Post-traumatic syndrome comprises irritability, anxiety and depression and it is associated with mild head injury. It is not yet clear whether post-traumatic syndrome is organic or psychological (Jackson, 1988).

It should be remembered that the trauma will also have a far-reaching effect on those close to the client who will simultaneously be involved in their own grief processes relating to the loss. However, the pattern may not be the same and individuals may be at different stages. The client may have reached the stage of depression while the relative is still denying and trying to motivate the client to work hard at rehabilitation. Thus each may interfere with the other's grieving.

People with communication problems have much to come to terms with and professionals involved in their care must not underestimate the extent of the distress. Some clients never do adjust and all too frequently the medical care is thorough while the emotional problems are left untouched. Such clients have the additional problem in that, by the very nature of their disorder, they are not be able to verbalize their anxieties or initiate discussion about them, in which case others should be prepared to do so. However, it is often easier for clinicians to avoid raising the issues as this necessitates a certain amount of personal risk, not to mention time. It can be uncomfortable to acknowledge and face real distress in another person, touching as this does on our own fears and anxieties. Remembering our own experiences of loss and pain can be a good starting point. Particularly with a communication handicapped person, simply acknowledging his feelings without necessarily trying to solve any of his problems lessens his sense of isolation and can bring some relief.

10

Alternative and augmented communication

COMMUNICATION AIDS

In alternative and augmented communication (AAC), some devised system operates in place of, or as a supplement to, the natural one. The complexity of these varies from computers right through to picture charts. In alternative communication systems, the client's own communication channels are completely replaced by other techniques, whereas in augmented communication the client's existing communicative ability is enhanced and extended in some way. To benefit from either approach, the client and their family need to come to regard total communication as the goal and to accept that speech may or may not form a part of that system.

Communication aids are not a new concept, in fact the first recorded aid was an Egyptian one that relied on pebbles. Electronic artificial larynxes came on the market in the early part of this century and since then there has been a rapidly expanding market, particularly in electronic and computer devices.

Clients who have had normal communication and lost it are often resistant to the idea of supplementing their abilities with any gadget or system. They see this as something artificial and frequently view it as an admission of defeat by themselves and their rehabilitators. They do not appreciate the part that is normally played by other modalities in day-to-day interactions. A normal facility with communication has been lost and anything less than its full restoration feels like failure. For clients the point at which the issue of AAC is raised is psychologically very hard as it is the point at which they have to accept the realities of their situation. On the other hand, clients who are born with communication difficulties seem to view artificial aids much more as representing an expansion of their abilities rather than a contraction.

Even electronic aids are not a panacea. A piece of equipment cannot simply be picked up for the problem to be solved. Many commercially available aids need to be adapted for individuals and, even with the most sophisticated aids, communication is far slower and more laborious than when using intelligible speech. Most clients have to be trained to use even quite basic aids, as do their potential listeners.

There are many considerations to take into account when selecting an aid but choosing an appropriate signalling system and access to that system is vital. There is no point in using a system based on written words, such as a word processor or word chart, if the user has poor literacy skills, in which case he may be better off with pictures or Blissymbolics. Having decided which symbols are going to be used in place of spoken words the person has to have some means of selecting individual symbols and indicating that selection to others. For people with physical disabilities where motor movement is severely impaired, designing a suitable access to the symbols can be challenging. An AAC system can have many functions. It can enable an individual to regulate social interaction, obtain objects or bring about certain actions, transfer information, express emotion, express aspects of self, allow the recreational aspects of communication such as chatting and writing letters to occur and make sure that conversations are understood by both parties. It may not be possible to achieve all this with one item, so for example a person may need a buzzer to attract attention, a picture chart to interact with friends and an aid with some speech output for using with strangers on the telephone.

There are many AAC systems available but because the market changes so swiftly it is only possible to give an overview of the strategies underlying the different types.

Signing and manual gesture systems

There are several widely used systems. They are popularly thought of as only having application with the hearing impaired but they are also extensively used with dysarthric and dysphasic clients, people with learning difficulties and people with physical handicaps. Commonly used systems include British Sign Language,

American Sign Language, finger-spelling, Makaton, Amerind and Paget-Gorman. Signing systems require a level of manual dexterity (although some can be adapted for clients who only have the use of one hand) and an audience that knows or is willing to learn the signs. They can be used either in place of or to supplement existing speech.

Low-tech communication aids

In general these do not allow effective group participation unless accompanied by some other means of attracting attention. There is a wide range of such aids available and many can be assembled to fit specific requirements.

Hand-writing aids

For literate non-verbal individuals who have sufficient hand or foot control to write, this may be the most effective way of communicating. Aids that facilitate legible writing include pen grips, arm rests, paper holders and mountings for people in bed to enable them to write while lying down.

Picture charts

These are commonly used by stroke patients and people with learning difficulties. The person points to one of several pictures to indicate what they want. In practice this is limited to expressing basic needs. Often the most appropriate form for such a chart is a ring-bound file which can be easily carried. Such files can contain family pictures and biographical information so the person can give information about themselves to strangers. Photographs may be used in place of line drawings.

Symbol chart

The two most commonly used are Rebus for people with learning difficulties and Blissymbolics for the physically handicapped. In Blissymbolics the picture symbol is accompanied by a written word which enables a 'listener' who may be unfamiliar with the system to read the message. Both systems are dependent on a well motivated listener but, although they are helpful with expression, they do not cope well with such things as proper names.

Alphabet charts

These require the individual to spell out what they want to say letter by letter. It is a slow procedure but can be speeded up by omitting the vowels. Such charts need to include the words 'space', 'end' and 'error'.

Word charts

These can be built upon a single board or in a file and they consist of lists of words or phrases for the person to point to. It can be used in conjunction with an alphabet chart. This enables regularly used phrases to be given in full, with new phrases being spelt out. The various charts are usually accessed by the user pointing to the desired symbol, but if this is not possible there can be indirect access by a listener scanning the board with a finger until they reach the place the speaker wishes to be. The speaker indicates this by a pre-arranged signal such as nodding or vocalizing.

Eye-pointing and E-tran frames

Eye-blinking is another alternative for individuals who are unable to point accurately with their hands. A perspex sheet between the user and listener has written or picture items arranged round the edge. The user signals the target item by looking at it and the observer notes the direction of gaze. This system becomes less workable with large numbers of items.

High-tech aids

Most types of electronic aids are accessed through button or key presses. Indirect access can be achieved by a scanning system, usually a moving light which is halted at the correct item by activating a switch.

Speech support

Here the user's own speech is enhanced. Someone who has poor volume as in Parkinson's disease or when using oesophageal speech may need an amplifier to enable other people to hear them. A range of amplifiers are available and hand-held, throat or clip-on microphones can be selected to meet the user's need. It must be remembered that amplifiers amplify everything, so if there is imprecise articulation any inappropriate noise will be amplified as well. Amplifiers can be used to deal with noisy speaking situations.

A person who has no voice, for whatever reason, may wish to use an artificial larynx. These are about the size and shape of an electric shaver and a small head is made to vibrate by depressing a button. The head is held against the neck and the vibration is transmitted across the neck wall to set air inside the vocal tract in motion (Fig. 7.4). If articulation is superimposed on this vibrating air column, recognizable words are produced. This speech sounds like a synthesizer and lacks intonation but used skilfully it can be easily intelligible and takes less effort to produce than, say, oesophageal speech.

Scanning boards

Here sophisticated electronic scanning systems are used to select words, pictures, symbols or letters. They can be used by themselves or as an access to a computer such as a keyboard emulator which mimics a normal keyboard but the 'keys' are selected by using a switch to scan the keyboard.

Aids with written output

A written output can be obtained in the form of a printout. Such devices which were originally designed for the business market are usually small with some capacity for storing words and phrases. They are generally used with dysarthric patients and some people with cerebral palsy. With literate clients they are easy to learn to use but they do need one-to-one contact with a literate user to be effective.

Digitized speech output

These machines record real speech which is then accessed through pictures or written words via key presses or scanning. They have good intelligibility as they use human speech, but are limited in their storage capacity. They express basic needs but for more sophisticated expression are best used in conjunction with other systems. They enable group participation and use of the telephone.

Synthesized speech output

Direct access or scanning versions are available. The speech is generated by letter or picture/symbol selection. These devices permit the use of novel utterances and hence allow better interaction in group settings. However, it may take the listener some time to tune in to the sound of the synthesized speech. They are mainly used with people who have dysarthria, cerebral palsy or learning difficulties.

Portable computer systems

Word processing packages, word stores and text stores can be linked up to speech synthesizers or printers. They have most potential for literate users and tend to be used mainly by people with acquired disorders who are in employment.

There is now a large range of switches to enable indirect access to these systems, such as hand and foot pressure, suck-blow, eye movement and joy-stick switches. The development of sensor switches that are sensitive to minimal muscle activity means that an individual can access a communication aid even if he/she only has control of one muscle.

For many people the need for alternative communication systems is a temporary one, for example during recovery in intensive care. Even so, it is essential to reduce the client's anxiety and enable the exchange of information with medical staff. Those with resolving conditions may require an aid to facilitate communication during the recovery period. This may be the case after orofacial surgery, the acute phases of multiple sclerosis and during recovery after stroke. It is sensible to introduce the aid early in the client's recovery process rather than at the end of direct therapy input when it may be seen as implying failure. AAC systems are more generally considered as a long-term means of communication for people who need a replacement for verbal communication. They are all much slower than normal communication.

Supplying such an aid or series of aids can be a complex business and involve many professionals both in the assessment and provision of suitable equipment. The funding of communication aids, at least in the UK, remains a complex and often frustrating business with several different possible sources of funding. Some aids, such as artificial larynxes, are available on prescription, but this can vary depending on the area of the country in which the client is being treated.

COMMUNICATION AID CENTRES

In the UK there are now a number of Communication Aid Centres that house substantial banks of commercially available aids to which clients can be referred for a detailed assessment of their needs and a subsequent recommendation of suitable aids and access systems. In some cases engineers work in conjunction with communication therapists at the centres and are able to design and adapt aids to individual clients. Unfortunately clients may have to wait some time to be seen at such a centre. Particularly in the case of progressive disorders, where a client's needs may change throughout the course of the disease, the normal funding mechanisms sometimes move too slowly and clients may be unable to use an aid by the time they receive it. The pressure for easy access to aid centres continues and undoubtedly things have improved in the last ten years. New devices are being developed all the time and old ones refined. For some of the people who need them they become a vital part of everyday life, for others they are used only at certain times or in particular situations. Either way they can help clients regain some personal dignity and control. I always take some pleasure in the story of a colleague who gave a Canon Communicator to a severely dysarthric client. This machine is essentially a small hand-held typewriter that prints out the message on a very narrow ribbon of tape. The client's very first act was to send a 9-feet long letter of complaint about his food and accommodation to the hospital administrator.

References

Aaronson, A. (1985) *Clinical Voice Disorders*, 2nd edn, Thieme Inc., New York.

Argyle, M. (1983) *Bodily Communications*, Methuen and Co, London.

Arieti, A. (1981) *Understanding and Helping the Schizophrenic*, Pelican Books, London.

Baxter, R., Cohen, S. B. and Ylvisaker, M. (1985) Comprehensive cognitive assessment, in *Head Injury Rehabilitation; Children and Adolescents* (ed. M. Ylvisaker), College Hill Press, San Diego, California, pp. 247–75.

Broe, G. A., Akhtar, A. J., Andrews, G. R. *et. al.* (1976) Neurological disorders in the elderly. *Journal of Neurology, Neurosurgery and Psychiatry*, **39**, 362–6.

Bryan, K. L. (1989) *The Right Hemisphere Language Battery*, Far Communications, Kidworth.

Coates, J. (1986) *Women, Men and Language*, Longman, London and New York.

Coupland, N. (1980) Style shifting in a Cardiff work setting, *Language in Society*, **9**, 1–22.

Crystal, D. (1980) *Introduction to Language Pathology*, Arnold, London.

Dabul, B. (1979) *Aphasia Battery for Adults*. CC Publications Inc. USA.

Darley, F. L., Aaronson, A. E. and Brown, J. R. (1969) Differential diagnostic patterns of dysarthria, *Journal of Speech and Hearing Research*, **12**, 246–69.

Darley, F. L. (1975) *Examination for Motor Dysfunction in Motor Speech Disorders*. Saunders. Philadelphia.

Enderby, P. and Philipp, R. (1986) Speech and language handicap: towards knowing the size of the problem. *British Journal of Disorders of Communication*, **21**, 151–65.

Enderby, P., Wood, V. and Wade, D. (1987) *The Frenchay Aphasia Screening Test*, NFER-Nelson, London.

Enderby, P. (1983) *Dysarthria Assessment*. College-Hill Press, San Diego.

Freeman, R. D., Carbin, C. F. and Boese, R. J. (1981) *Can't Your Child Hear?*, Croom Helm, London.

Gravell, R. (1988) *Communication Problems in Elderly People*, Croom Helm, London.

Goodglass, H. and Kaplan, E., (1983) *Boston Diagnostic Aphasia Examination*. Lea and Febiger, Phildelphia.

Jackson, H. (1988) Brain cognition and grief. *Aphasiology*, **2** (1), 89–92.

Kolvin, I. and Fundudis, T. (1981) Elective mutism in children. *Journal of Child Psychology and Psychiatry*, **22** (3), 219–32.

Lancer, J., Syder, D., Jones, A. S. and Le Boutillier, A. (1988) The outcome of different management patterns for vocal nodules. *Journal of Laryngology and Otology*, **102**.

Morris, D. (1981) *The Pocket Guide to Manwatching*, Triad Grafton, London.

McKenna, P. and Warrington, E. (1983) *Graded Naming Test*. NFER-Nelson, Windsor, England.

Oates, J. M. and Dacakis, G. (1983) Speech pathology considerations in the management of transexualism. *British Journal of Disorders of Communication*, **18** (3), 139–51.

Pease, A. (1981) *Body Language*, Sheldon Press, London.

Robertson, S., (1982) *Dysarthria Profile*, Robertson, Essex, UK.

Rollin, W. J. (1987) *The Psychology of Communication Disorders in Individuals and their Families*, Prentice-Hall, Inc., New Jersey.

Scott, S., Caird, F. I. and Williams, F. O. (1985) *Communication in Parkinson's Disease*, Croom Helm, London.

Schuell, H., (1973) *Differential Diagnosis of Aphasia with the Minnesota Test*, 2nd edn. University of Minnesota, Minneapolis.

Selby, G. (1968) Parkinson's disease, in *Handbook of Clinical Neurology*, vol. 6, (eds P. J. Vinken and G. W. Bray), North Holland Publishing Company, Amsterdam.

Syder, D., Body, R., Parker, M. and Boddy, M., (in press) *The Sheffield Screening Test for Acquired Language Disorders*. NFER-Nelson. Windsor, England.

Tanner, D. C. and Gerstenberger, D. L., (1988) The grief response to neuropathologies of speech and language. *Aphasiology*, **12** (1), 79–84.

Wheldall, K., Mittler, P. and Hobsbaum, A. (1979) *Sentence Comprehension Test*. NFER-Nelson, Windsor, England.

Whurr, R. (1974) *An Aphasia Screening Test*. R. Whurr, London.

Wolff, C. (1977) *Bisexuality, A Study*, Quartet Books, London.

Ylvisaker, M. and Szekeres, S. F, (1986) Management of the patient with closed head injury, in *Language Intervention Strategies in Adult Aphasia*, 2nd edn. (ed. R. Chappey), Williams and Wilkins, Baltimore, pp. 474–90.

Index